Nourish

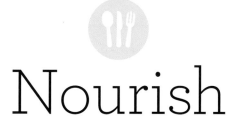

Nourish

Whole Food Recipes featuring Seeds, Nuts & Beans

BY NETTIE CRONISH AND CARA ROSENBLOOM, RD

whitecap

Whitecap Books is known for its expertise in the cookbook market, and has produced some of the most innovative and familiar titles found in kitchens across North America. Visit our website at www.whitecap.ca.

EDITOR: Jordie Yow
DESIGN: Maxine Matishak
FOOD PHOTOGRAPHY: Mike McColl
PROOFREADER: Lara Kordic

Printed in China

Library and Archives Canada Cataloguing in Publication

Cronish, Nettie, 1954-, author   Nourish : whole food recipes featuring seeds, nuts and beans / Nettie Cronish and Cara Rosenbloom.

ISBN 978-1-77050-243-7 (paperback)

   1. Cooking (Seeds). 2. Cooking (Nuts). 3. Cooking (Beans). 4. Cookbooks. I. Rosenbloom, Cara, 1974-, author II. Title.

TX814.5.S44C76 2015   641.6'56   C2015-905216-5

We acknowledge the financial support of the Government of Canada, and the Province of British Columbia through the Book Publishing Tax Credit.

Canadä

15 16 17 18 19 5 4 3 2 1

To my husband, Jim, and children, Cameron, Mackenzie and Emery. My essential beans and seeds. —Nettie

To my mom, who taught me how to cook with love. And to my dad, who at age 83 continues to teach me to live life fully, laugh daily and leave room for pastries. —Cara

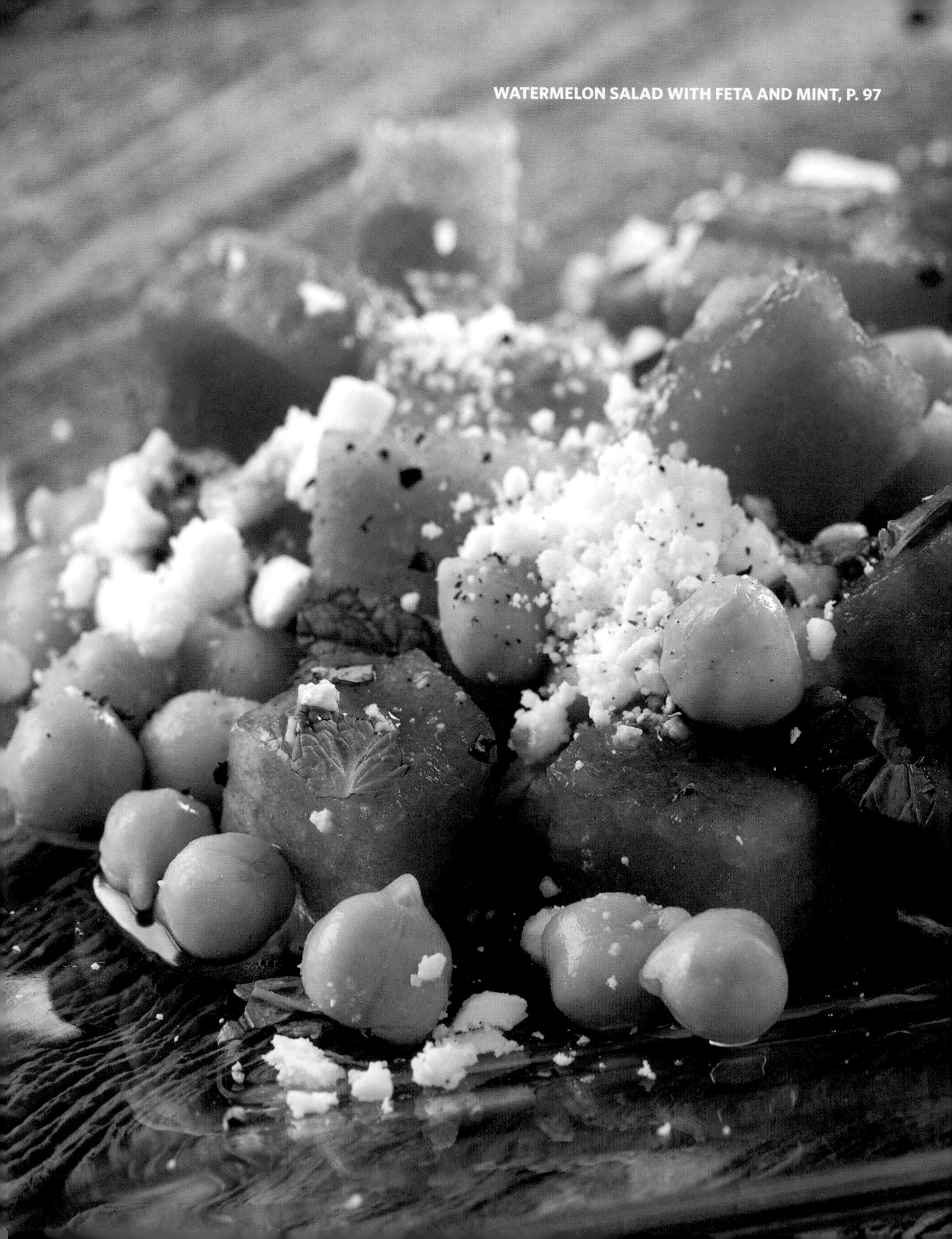

WATERMELON SALAD WITH FETA AND MINT, P. 97

Contents

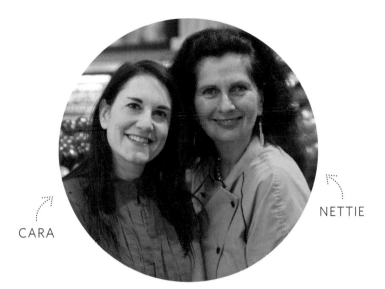

CARA

NETTIE

Introduction

ABOUT THE BOOK

Cara: Every time we met, Nettie and I inevitably discussed food. We found we shared a mutual adoration for vegetarian protein sources like beans, lentils, nuts and seeds. That's where this book was born. We wanted to pay homage to these nutrient-dense plant foods that are underutilized in most diets but are so good for you! We set out to create a book that has a bean, nut or seed in every recipe but still includes familiar foods. It's our way of infusing the goodness of these whole foods into the diet by introducing them to foods you already enjoy.

While the book is filled with many vegetarian ingredients, it's not a vegetarian cookbook. We both live in households with meat eaters, so we wanted them to love the recipes too. Meat, chicken, fish and seafood all make an appearance alongside vegetarian and vegan recipes—so there is something for everyone!

And the best news? An eating plan that's based on whole, unprocessed food is the recommended diet for preventing obesity, heart disease, high cholesterol, dementia, cancer, hypertension, diabetes and other health concerns that may be on your mind. Eating real food made from recognizable ingredients is great for whole body health!

Our hope is that this book gets you into the kitchen to cook. These recipes use nutritious whole food ingredients. With every bite, you're making better choices for a healthier lifestyle.

HOW THIS BOOK CAME TO BE

Nettie: I first met Cara six years ago at a Women's Culinary Network meeting. This network is an organization of culinary professionals, and we organize events themed around food. I was introduced to Cara, a culinary dietitian, as a new member who specialized in educating the public about healthy eating. But Cara was no ordinary dietitian. She is a passionate gourmand who cooks daily and follows the latest food trends.

Cara gave me a huge smile and asked me half a dozen questions about sourcing and cooking ingredients central to my vegetarian diet. I felt respected, appreciated and thankful. Here was a person I could work with and learn from.

Coming from a vegetarian, plant-based perspective, I come across a lot of alternative dietary information that makes health claims without any merit. Being able to reach out to Cara for her expertise and knowledge has made me a better chef and culinary instructor, and allows me to share ingredient information with a nutritional focus based on fact and not popular opinion.

When the opportunity came to write my next book, I knew that Cara was the right partner. We wanted to balance the culinary perspective with a sprinkling of nutrition, and ensure there was no junk or bunk. Everything is evidence-based, and because of Cara's background in communication, it's not overly scientific or complicated. It's actually fun, and I've learned so much from her over the past year.

Cara: Running my own business from a home office is rather isolating, so I am always looking for networking opportunities to meet like-minded foodies. When I stumbled upon the Women's Culinary Network, I immediately joined and began attending their events. I met the network chair, Nettie Cronish, and what I liked about her was her ability to engage anyone in very interesting conversation, and then pull others into the chat, continuously making connections and introductions. My contact list grew exponentially after just one event.

When Nettie asked me if I'd like to collaborate on her next book, I did not hesitate! I have always loved to cook, and I knew that I would learn so much about recipe development and testing by working with a published cookbook author. And that's precisely what happened.

Nettie and I spent a year developing and testing recipes along with Heather Howe, a professional home economist, recipe tester and cooking instructor. What a perfect fit Heather was to our team! Nettie knew her from a past job, and I knew her from our overlapping time at *Canadian Living* magazine. Plus, since Nettie is vegetarian and I eat fish and seafood but no meat, Heather was also our professional taster for dishes that contained meat or poultry.

The three of us worked harmoniously to plate 12 dishes in a typical eight-hour work day, breaking for lunch to taste and evaluate our creations. There were many mishaps, lots of "Wow—that's amazing!" exclamations, tons of storytelling and loads of laughter. Food brings people together. Both of these amazing women have taught me so much about cooking and embracing food. I am forever grateful for this experience.

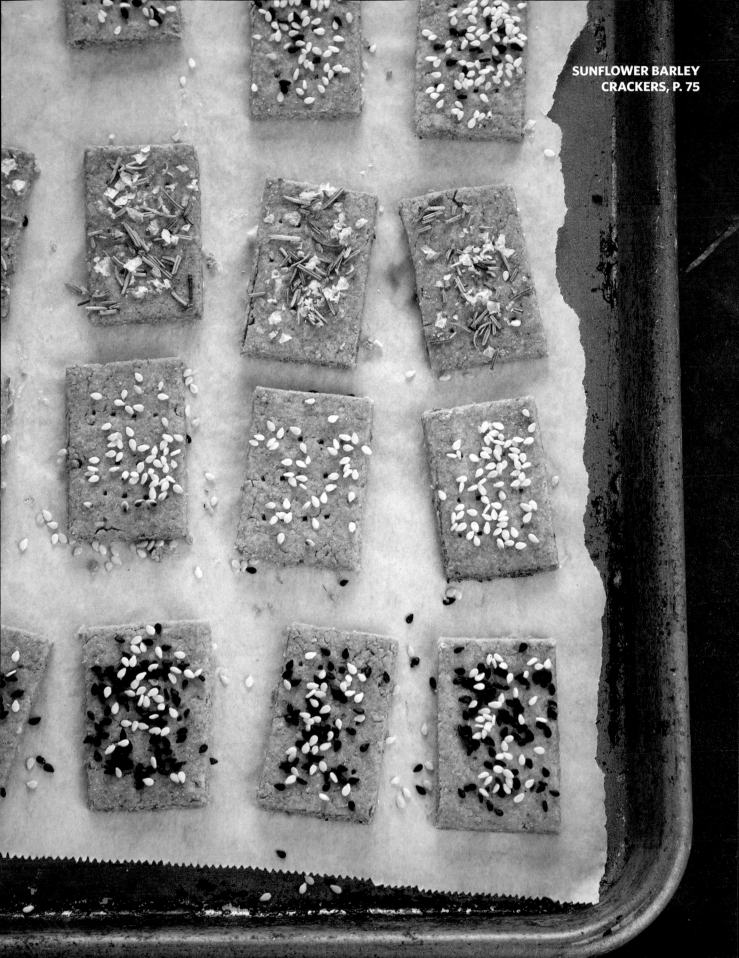

SUNFLOWER BARLEY CRACKERS, P. 75

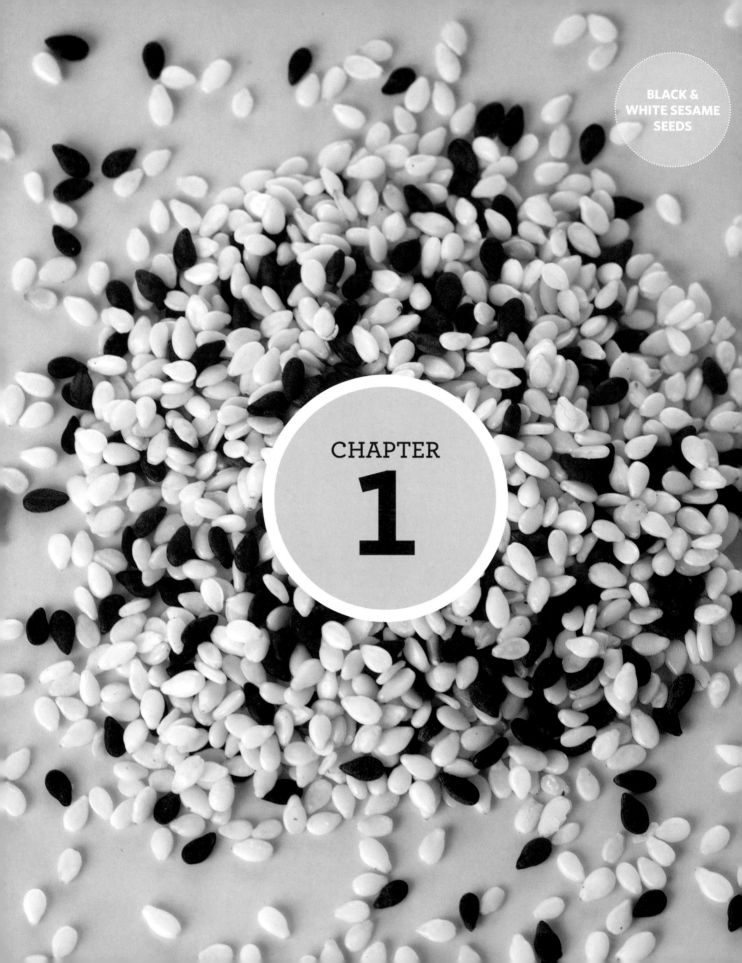

BLACK &
WHITE SESAME
SEEDS

CHAPTER

1

Nutrition Quick & Simple

BY CARA ROSENBLOOM

I've been a registered dietitian for 15 years, so this introduction to nutrition could easily be about the nutrient needs of the human body. But it won't be. Explaining exact numbers for the grams of protein or calcium you need each day is impractical and hard to follow. So let's skip it.

Instead, I'd like to share the words that changed the way I think about food and nutrients, and significantly altered the way I practise as a dietitian and educate others about nutrition. It was at the 2006 Dietitians of Canada National Conference in Halifax, Nova Scotia, in a session featuring dietitians who were also chefs—Gerry Kasten and Mary Sue Waisman.

At that lecture, Mary Sue eloquently explained that "people eat food, not nutrients." And it stuck with me. Until that moment, I (and every dietitian I knew) was trained to provide nutrient information. But suddenly, instead of recommending that someone needed 300 mg of calcium, I was going to suggest a morning latte instead (a delicious way to get 300 mg of calcium!) So simple, and such a huge change. The emphasis I placed on food had been missing, and I needed to get back to it to truly inspire people to eat better.

That one sentence changed the way I saw food. While food nourishes, it's not about counting grams of fibre. It's about the experience of flavour. It's about dining with friends and family. It's about cooking and transforming ingredients into meals. It's about enjoyment.

If I wrote this book as a newly trained dietitian, the words "folate" and "potassium" and "magnesium" may have filled this nutritional overview, because I was educated about nutrients. And while those nutrients are crucial for health, it's unlikely that you eat pizza for the calcium or enjoy bananas for the potassium. We eat what tastes good.

So, instead of nutritional minutia, let's look at the big picture. Let's embrace food for its potential to nourish us while we enjoy it. In the next few pages—and in 100 recipes—I'm going to tell you what I cook, what I eat and why I love it.

COOKING AT HOME: A SMALL PEP TALK

"Plan ahead, keep menus simple, and use lots of canned, packaged and frozen foods."
—L. Chapman, *Good Housekeeping*, 1950

Wow, has that advice ever changed over the last 65 years! Quick-to-prepare and processed foods really took off in the 1950s as a way to bring convenience to our lives. But in the present day, we know it is healthiest to cook with fresh, whole ingredients and shy away from processed foods. That's how I've set up my kitchen and my lifestyle.

Back in the 1950s, we didn't know the harm that processed foods could potentially have, especially if we ate too much of them. We now know that the combination of excess salt, cheap fats, refined flour, sugar, food colouring and preservatives is a very unhealthy mix. The shift is to cook from scratch more often, skipping the processed foods.

Last year I was fortunate to attend a lecture by food journalist Michael Pollan to support his book *Cooked*, which encourages us to "eat anything you want, as long as you cook it yourself." His take-home message was clear: cooking is the best way to stay healthy.

Many of my fellow dietitians agree. Registered dietitian and *National Post* columnist Jennifer Sygo cites cooking as one of the big food trends for 2015. She explains that during the past 50 years people have been fixated on convenient alternatives like fast food, processed products and ready-made items that are more like science experiments than food. She concludes that "we would be better served by spending more of our energy on learning how to prepare healthful whole foods at home, and less time counting grams of fibre or fat on prepackaged food from the grocery store."

LET'S GET COOKING!

New York Times food columnist Mark Bittman says it would be wonderful to "get people to see cooking as a joy rather than a burden." And cooking can be joyful. There is something therapeutic in the rhythmic slicing, dicing, stirring and whirring that takes place as you turn raw ingredients into something delicious.

Cooking is also filled with pressures—time, planning, cost, cleaning up and, of course, the burden of pleasing others. That's not always easy if the chairs at the table are filled by a group of people with diverse palates. I cook most days and am not immune to these challenges! But cooking does not need to be complicated or stressful.

Your definition of cooking may be as simple as boiling pasta. But with a handful of cherry tomatoes and some Parmesan, you've got dinner in 15 minutes! That's great! Or perhaps you have more sophisticated cooking skills, and are comfortable with a chef's knife and a mandolin. That's also great. The goal is to rely less on processed food and spend more time in the kitchen, in whichever way you can accomplish that feat. Not complicated or stressful.

The good news as I see it? Statistics show that Canadian home cooks are busy, preparing breakfast and lunch at home five days a week and dinner six days a week. Almost 70 percent of us make dinner at home, so the shift towards cooking is slowly happening.

The question is, what are we preparing? That's where the problem may lie. The study of what Canadians eat is so wide that it could fill a whole book. And while about 25 percent of Canadians are thought to be health-conscious and about 50 percent are more ingredient-conscious, the remaining 25 percent are not engaged in healthy eating at all. And because of that diversity, what we prepare has a huge range. When we cook at home using processed ingredients, are we really cooking?

The top meals cooked at home are usually pasta dishes, chicken, vegetables, casseroles and fish. How healthy these are depends on the ingredients that are used to make them. And that, of course, depends on what you buy at the grocery store, which is where the foundation of healthy cooking begins.

SHOP FOR A HEALTHY KITCHEN

The foods you purchase will influence the recipes you make, and whatever is in the fridge and pantry is what will go into your meals. So, the key to healthy eating is twofold:

1. Shop for nutritious ingredients.
2. Cook nourishing recipes. (We have put 100 of them into your hands!)

You can use the grocery list on page 10 to stock your kitchen with the right ingredients to prepare healthy and nutritious meals. I like to group them into three categories, and really highlight the difference between packaged foods and processed foods:

Whole foods

These foods are as close to nature as they can be. They have not been highly altered, and no further ingredients have been added to them. Examples are vegetables, fruit, dry beans, whole grains, nuts, seeds, fish and poultry. These are the best foods for your body and your mind. A diet based in whole foods can help reduce the risk of heart disease, type 2 diabetes, dementia and some types of cancer. Fill your cart with these foods first.

Packaged foods

Foods may be sold in boxes or bags as the most convenient way to get them home from the store. And many of these foods have health benefits and can help make cooking more convenient—a double win! Packaged foods have been slightly altered from the way they appear in nature, but the changes have not reduced their health value. They are different than processed foods (see definition below). And while packaged foods may contain some minor additional ingredients, they are not detrimental to our health. Examples include: whole grain pasta, no-salt-added canned beans, tomato paste and tofu. Use these foods to complement the whole foods in your cart.

Processed foods

These items have been radically changed from how they once appeared in nature. They may be highly refined, which means they are processed to a new consistency that often eliminates the once valuable vitamins, minerals or fibre that the food contained. They may contain food colouring and preservatives, or they may have excess salt, sugar, trans fat or other undesirable nutrients that can lead to chronic disease when consumed in excess. Examples include candy, soda, deli meats, cookies, chips, crackers, cereals, condiments and sauces. For healthy eating, these items should not be the foundation of your grocery cart or your kitchen.

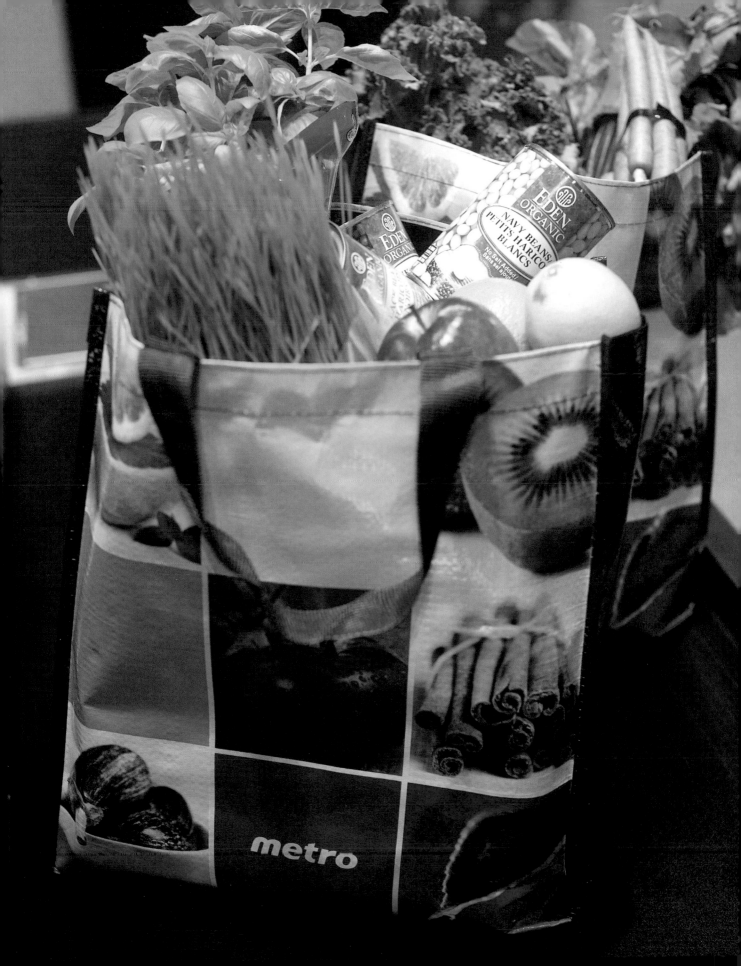

YOUR HEALTHY GROCERY LIST

Your healthy kitchen starts at the grocery store. Bring home the right ingredients to make cooking easier! This list contains the basics necessities that you'd find in my pantry and the key ingredients we used in this book. It's not an exhaustive list—sometimes you will need a specific ingredient for a particular recipe, so review your recipe before you shop. All of these items are whole or packaged foods; none are processed.

PRODUCE SECTION

- Fruit: berries, apples, pears, kiwis, bananas, oranges, lemons, limes, etc.
- Vegetables: carrots, celery, tomatoes, cucumbers, kale, chard, sweet peppers, broccoli, etc.
- Fresh herbs: parsley, cilantro, basil, mint, dill
- Organic tofu

BULK

- Nuts: almonds, walnuts, pecans, pistachios, pine nuts, cashews
- Seeds: chia, flax, sesame, pumpkin, sunflower, hemp
- Unsweetened dried fruit: raisins, apricots, cherries, cranberries
- Peanuts

FRESH

As needed:

- Chicken, fish, lamb, beef, seafood, etc.
- Whole grain breads

PANTRY STAPLES

- No-salt-added canned beans
- Dried lentils
- Canned tuna and salmon
- Whole grain pasta
- Brown rice
- Quinoa
- Millet
- Amaranth
- Large flake oats
- Flours: whole grain wheat, spelt, barley, oat, quinoa
- Nut and seed butters: almond, cashew, peanut, tahini
- No-salt-added broth

CONDIMENTS

- Extra virgin olive oil
- Toasted sesame oil
- Sodium-reduced tamari
- Vinegars: Balsamic, apple cider, rice wine, red wine
- Dijon mustard

DAIRY/EGGS

- Plain 2% Greek yogurt
- Milk (skim, 1% or 2%)
- Fortified soy beverage
- Cheddar, mozzarella, Parmesan and feta cheese
- Eggs
- Unsalted butter

FROZEN

- Fruit: mango, peaches and assorted berries
- Vegetables: peas, organic corn, broccoli
- Edamame

HERBS AND SPICES

- Basil
- Cinnamon
- Cardamom
- Ginger
- Nutmeg
- Garam masala
- Curry powder
- Oregano
- Thyme

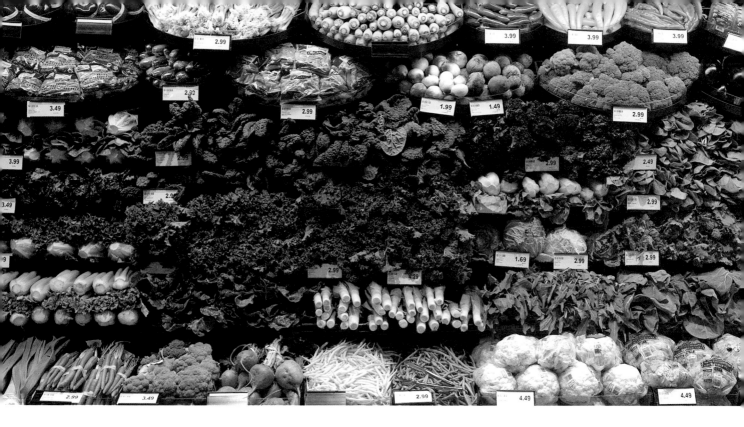

DON'T BELIEVE THE HYPE

As you build your healthy fridge and pantry, you will notice that there is a wide variety of nutritious foods to choose from. It's always good to remember that there is no one superfood that you should eat for optimal health, and that wellness comes from balance. No matter how popular kale, acai berries or almond milk become, one ingredient alone is not enough for your best health. Eating a kale salad before your triple bacon cheeseburger and poutine does not make the overall meal healthier!

Every week there seems to be a new study that claims to have found the answer to the problem of our unhealthy North American diet. Obesity, heart disease, diabetes and cancer are routinely blamed on food. It's sugar. No, it's genetically modified foods. Nope, it's gluten. Uh-uh. It's high-fructose corn syrup. No way. It's refined white flour. No, really, it's trans fat.

The truth is, no one food causes all of these health problems on its own. A constant unhealthy eating pattern, followed day after day, combined with inactivity, is what causes the most harm. The influence of our environment, individual genetics, education level and socio-economic status also come into play. It's a complex web.

Collectively, if you look at all of the culprits that are being blamed for North America's current health crisis—white flour, sugar, salt, GMO crops, fake fat—they are all found in abundance in one place: processed foods. If you cut back on refined, processed foods with many ingredients and stick to more natural whole food choices, you can effortlessly avoid all of the "baddies" that come along with the sealed bag or box.

Keep it simple, choose foods close to nature and cook when you can.

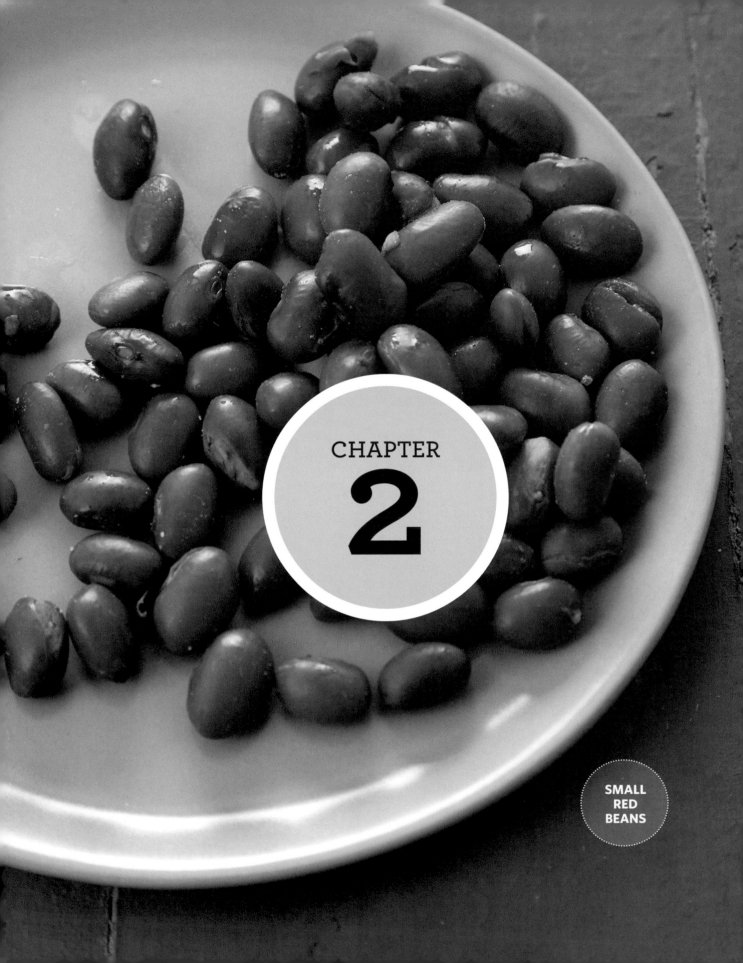

CHAPTER

2

SMALL
RED
BEANS

The Power of Seeds, Nuts & Beans

This book started as a way to capitalize on our mutual love for beans, nuts and seeds, in the hopes of encouraging others to include more of these versatile ingredients in their diet. Underutilized and über-healthy, they are the most overlooked foods in the kitchen. To promote their use, every recipe in this book will contain a bean, nut or seed.

Sometimes these ingredients are combined with cheese, meat, poultry, fish or seafood, and sometimes they are the stand-alone protein for the meal. Versatile, nutritious and delicious, they can be used—as you will see—in everything from appetizers to soups to desserts.

A BIT ABOUT LEGUMES

Beans, peas and lentils, and other legumes, are the edible seeds that grow in pods of plants. A good source of protein and iron, legumes are a healthy substitute for meat.

Cuisines from all over the world use legumes in many ways, from Indian lentil dal to Mexican black bean burritos to Mediterranean chickpea hummus. In addition to their cross-cultural uses and wide versatility, they have many health benefits too. High in fibre, they are an asset for managing blood cholesterol and blood sugar levels.

Legumes are sold fresh, dried or canned. We chose to use canned beans for most of the recipes in this book for one very important reason: convenience. Canned beans are pre-cooked and ready to use once opened, thus skipping the long process of soaking and cooking dried beans.

But, we chose our canned beans carefully and used Eden Foods beans because they have no salt added and the cans do not contain Bisphenol A (BPA) in the can lining. An industrial chemical, BPA is used to make the epoxy resin that lines cans, and may possibly migrate into the food. Exposure to BPA has been linked with some negative health effects, especially in children. And while most

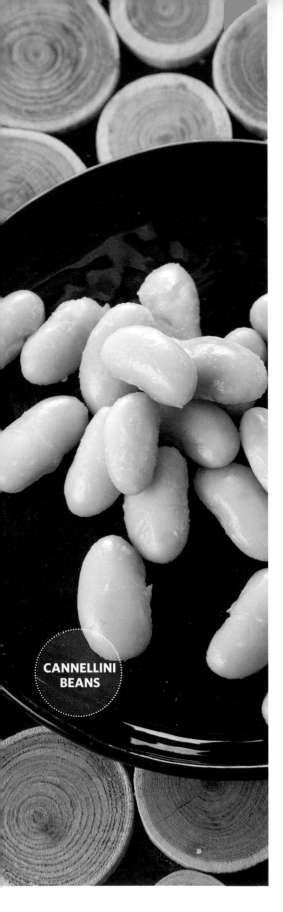

CANNELLINI BEANS

of us don't take in enough BPA to cause harm, if a BPA-free alternatives are available, it makes sense to use them.

Some canned beans can have up to 1,000 mg of sodium per cup, which is a very high amount considering your body only requires 1,500 mg of sodium in the entire day. We chose beans with no added salt, so you can control the sodium content and overall flavour of your dish. We give control to you, the home cook.

The other great thing about Eden Foods beans is that they are cooked and canned with kombu, a type of seaweed. Cooking beans with seaweed helps break down the flatulence-causing component of beans, so they are easier to digest and cause less gas. And, yeah, that's important!

If time permits, you can certainly cook beans from scratch. The quickest way is to use a pressure cooker, but the old-fashioned stovetop method works too (it just takes longer).

Tip: Freezing Beans

If you've soaked and cooked more beans than you need, you can freeze the leftovers. Allow the cooked beans to cool, and store beans in large plastic containers with tight fitting lids, or in freezer bags. Label the type of bean and the date you cooked them. Beans can be frozen for up to six months. To thaw your beans for use in salads or other cold dishes, defrost them in the fridge for a day. If you are making soup, stew or other cooked dishes, you can use beans straight from the freezer.

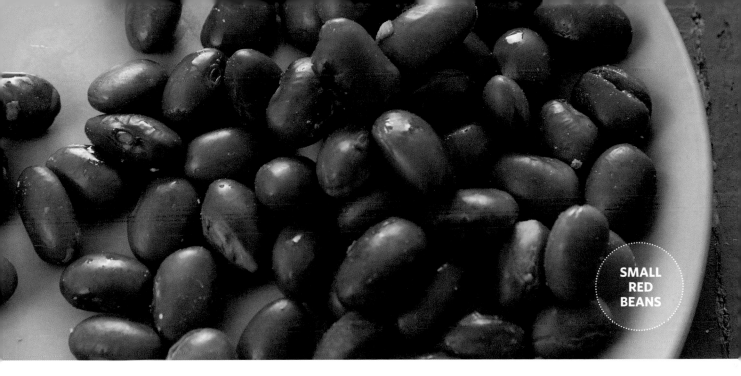

HOW TO BUY, SOAK AND COOK BEANS FROM SCRATCH

Buy: Beans last a long time, but older beans take longer to cook. Packaged dried beans may have helpful expiry dates, but bulk beans probably do not. If buying in bulk, purchase your beans at a store where they are sold and restocked often. Choose beans that are bright in colour and uniform in shape, and avoid packaged beans that are discolored, chipped, split, cracked or have a musty smell.

Soak: Save cooking time by soaking your dried beans first. Bonus: soaking beans helps reduce the starches that cause unpleasant gas and bloating. Never cook your beans in their soaking water; it contains the indigestible natural sugars that cause gas.

The traditional soak method

1. Sort beans. Discard any stones or debris. Rinse beans.
2. Pour cold water over beans to cover.
3. Soak beans per times listed on the chart on the opposite page.
4. Drain and discard water used for soaking. Rinse with fresh, cool water.

The quick soak method

1. Sort beans. Discard any stones or debris. Rinse beans.
2. Place beans in a large pot and add 6 cups of water for every 2 cups of beans.
3. Bring to boil for 3 minutes.
4. Remove beans from heat, cover, and let stand for 1 hour.
5. Drain and discard water used for soaking. Rinse with fresh, cool water.

Cook: Cooking times for beans varies depending on the size and age of the beans. Remember to add a strip of kombu seaweed to help break down the starch that contains gas. Kombu is sold in packages in health food stores (it's a 4 x 1 inch/10 x 2.5 cm black rectangle that softens in water). The chart below has helpful cooking times. In general, you add 2 cups (500 mL) of cold water for every cup of soaked bean, bring to a boil, lower heat and simmer, partially covered per these cooking times:

LEGUME NAME	CHARACTERISTICS	SOAKING TIME	COOKING TIME	PRESSURE COOKER
Aduki beans	Small, dark red beans used in traditional Japanese cuisine.	4 hours	1–1.5 hours	20 minutes
Black beans	Small, plump kidney-shaped beans with a shiny black-blue coat and an earthy flavour.	4 hours	1–1.5 hours	20 minutes
Black-eyed peas	Small white beans with a characteristic black dot.	4 hours	1–1.5 hours	20 minutes
Chickpeas	Small, round, beige legumes. Also called garbanzo beans.	8 hours or overnight	1.5–2 hours	20 minutes
Fava beans	Also known as broad beans, they are large in size and have a creamy texture.	8 hours or overnight	1.5–2 hours	25 minutes
Kidney beans	Long, kidney-shaped legumes found red or white (white also called cannellini beans).	8 hours or overnight	1.5–2 hours	25 minutes
Pinto beans	Oval-shaped beans with speckled coats ranging from brown to cranberry red.	8 hours or overnight	1.5–2 hours	20 minutes
Small red beans	Similar to red kidney beans, but half the size.	8 hours or overnight	1–1.5 hours	20 minutes

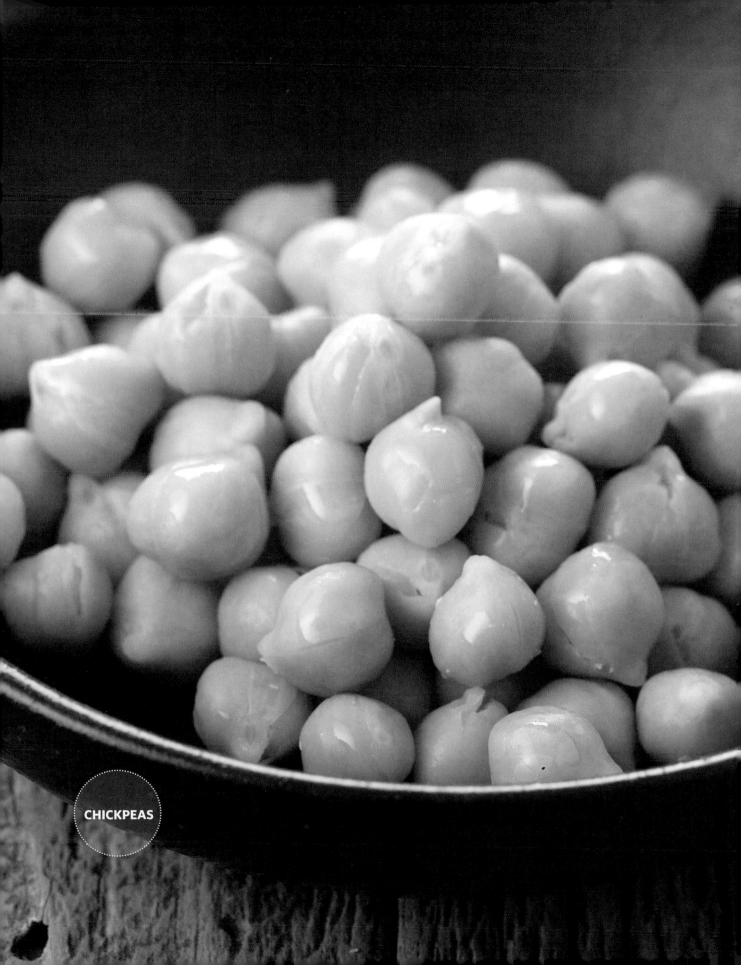

CHICKPEAS

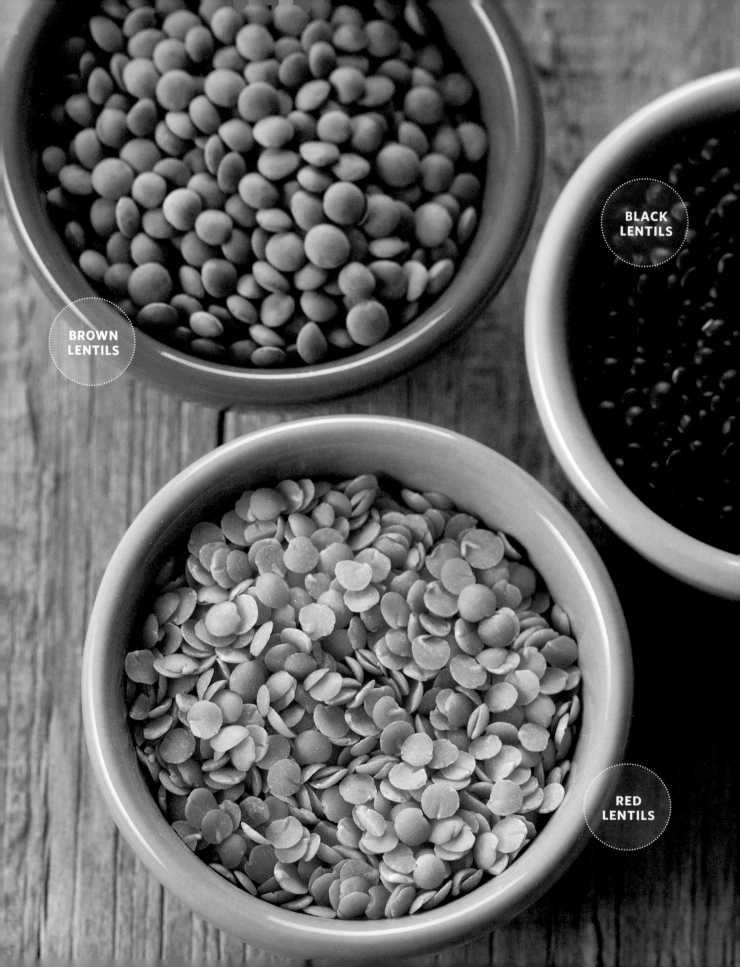

BLACK
LENTILS

BROWN
LENTILS

RED
LENTILS

LENTILS

A cousin to peas and beans, lentils are also legumes. They are smaller and more convenient since they do not need to be pre-soaked, and they cook more quickly than peas and beans. In this cookbook, lentils were cooked from scratch, since they take just 15–35 minutes (depending on the type of lentil) and do not require pre-soaking before they are prepared. Pressure cookers are not recommended for cooking lentils.

How to cook lentils from scratch

1. Sort to discard stones or debris.

2. No soaking is required! Rinse in a sieve under cool running water.

3. Boil per the instructions on the chart:

LEGUME NAME	CHARACTERISTICS	LENTIL: WATER RATIO	COOKING TIME
Black, green and brown lentils	Small, disc-shaped legumes that retain their shape when cooked.	1 cup (250mL): 2½ cups (625mL)	25–35 minutes
Red lentils	Peeled, split orange-coloured lentils that do not hold their shape when cooked; they become creamy.	1 cup (250mL): 2 cups (500mL)	15–25 minutes

Note: It is important to use unsalted water since salt toughens the lentils, making them take longer to cook.

SOY

The versatile soybean is also a legume, but it gets special mention because it's the starting point for so many other foods, such as tofu, tempeh and fortified soy beverages. This complete protein is the closest vegetarian alternative to meat.

We use these soy products in the book:

Tofu

Sometimes called bean curd, tofu is a white, neutral-tasting soy food. To make tofu, soybeans are soaked, drained, ground, strained, simmered and then pressed to different consistencies. It's available in a range from extra firm to silken (soft). Leftover tofu can be frozen for a maximum of six months. It must be defrosted before use.

Fortified Soy Beverage

This is the fluid that comes from pressed soybeans. Fortified or enriched versions contain calcium, vitamin D and other nutrients to make them nutritionally equivalent to cow's milk.

Edamame

Smooth green soybeans in the pod. They are available fresh or frozen, shelled or in the pod.

Tempeh

A high-protein cultured food made from soybeans and grains. Invented in Indonesia, tempeh is traditionally made by culturing cooked, cracked soybeans with the mold *Rhizopus oligosporus*. The fermentation process enhances the flavour and makes soybeans easier to digest. Tempeh has a firm, chewy texture and a mild, mushroom-like taste.

A Note About Tamari

We use good quality tamari, which is similar to soy sauce but contains no (or much less) wheat. Tamari is a traditional Japanese condiment made from fermented soybeans. Soy sauce is traditionally Chinese, and is made by cooking soybeans with roasted wheat and other grains in a 50:50 ratio. Tamari has a darker colour and richer flavour, with less of a salty bite. We specifically use sodium-reduced tamari with 25 percent less sodium than "regular" tamari.

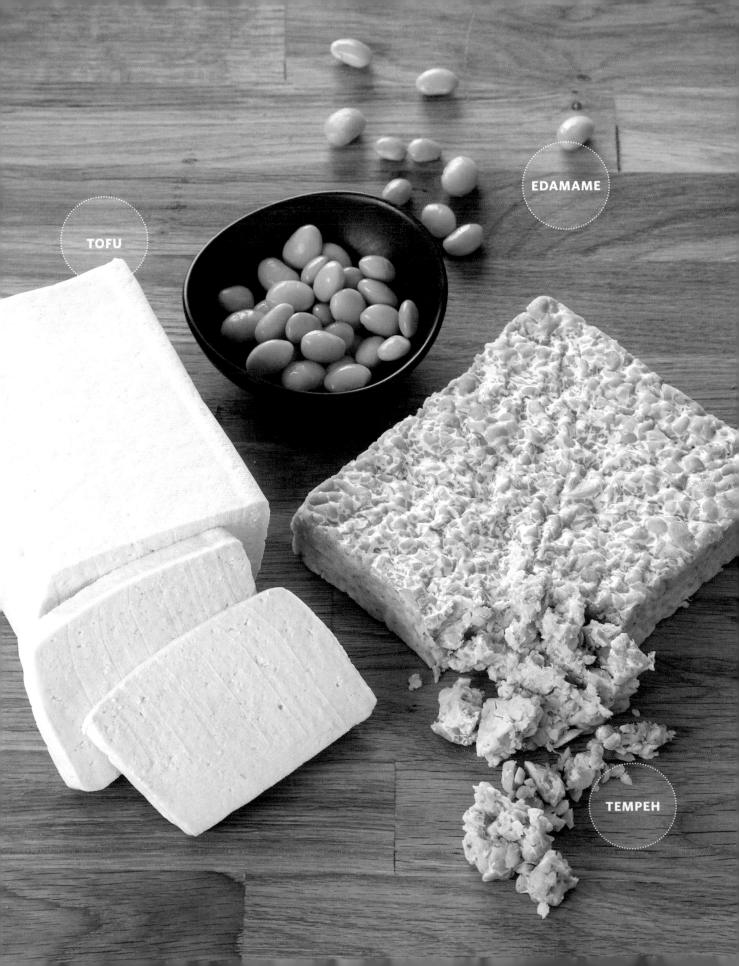

TOFU

EDAMAME

TEMPEH

NUTS

The research on the health benefits of nuts is simply outstanding. For each daily serving of nuts, the risk of developing heart disease drops by almost 30 percent. Think about that for a second. You just need to eat ¼ cup (60 mL) of nuts (about the amount that would fill a shot glass!) to reap this amazing protective benefit. The studies show eating nuts just four times a week can have these stellar health benefits, though you can eat them every day if you prefer.

Remember, because nuts have about 160–200 calories per ¼ cup (60 mL) serving, they need to be eaten instead of another snack, not in addition to it.

Which nut should you have? As the chart shows, each nut is high in a different nutrient. That means eating mixed nuts is ideal if you want to get a range of different vitamins, minerals and other healthy compounds, and the heart health benefits have been shown with all of these nuts. Nut butters are also fantastic!

NUT NAME	CHARACTERISTICS	HEALTH BENEFITS
Almonds	Off-white in colour, covered by a thin brownish skin. Shelled almonds are available whole, sliced or slivered, either with their skin or blanched with skin removed.	Highest in protein, calcium, fibre and vitamin E.
Cashews	C-shaped, fleshy tropical tree fruits that are enclosed in a tough shell. They have a buttery, mellow flavour.	Highest in vitamin K, iron and zinc.
Peanuts	Actually legumes and not nuts, these small bites come two or three to a shell and can be eaten plain or roasted.	Highest in folate and niacin.
Pecans	Brown, bumpy nuts that come from inside a smooth, oval-shaped shell.	Highest in antioxidants.
Pine nuts	Small seeds from pine cones of evergreen trees. They are also called pignolias.	Highest in manganese.
Pistachios	A hard, cream-coloured exterior shell holds the light green seed inside, which is covered in purple-brown papery skin.	Highest in potassium, vitamin B_6 and thiamin.
Walnuts	Two off-white bumpy lobes that look like abstract butterflies, covered in a thin, light brown skin. English walnuts are the most common.	Highest in omega-3 fat.

SEEDS

Technically, legumes and nuts are also seeds in the botanical sense—but for our purposes, we're sticking with the culinary use of the word seeds: sesame, pumpkin, sunflower and the like. This is also where we will categorize grain-like seeds such as quinoa, amaranth and millet.

SEED NAME	CHARACTERISTICS	HEALTH BENEFITS
Amaranth	A tiny yellow seed from flowering plants. It has a gelatinous quality, similar to oatmeal, when cooked.	Very high in phosphorus and manganese; source of fibre.
Chia	Tiny ovals that can be black, white or multi-hued. They have a mild, nutty flavour.	Source of fibre, protein, omega-3 fat, magnesium and phosphorus. Contains antioxidants.
Flax	Small, brown or light beige tear-shaped seeds. They are a good replacement for eggs in baking. Use ground flax to release the nutrients inside the seed coat.	Source of omega-3 fats, fibre, thiamin and antioxidant lignans.
Hemp	Hemp seeds have a pleasant, mild flavour. While hemp is a species of cannabis, it is not the same as marijuana and has no psychoactive compounds.	High in protein, potassium and omega-3 fats.
Millet	Small, round yellow seeds. Served as a side dish, similar to rice, it cooks up fluffy with a mildly nutty flavour.	Source of magnesium and fibre.
Pumpkin	Also known as pepitas, these are the edible green seeds that grow inside the outer white seed coat in pumpkins. Mildly flavoured, they pop when toasted, so stand back.	Source of manganese, magnesium, phosphorus and zinc.
Quinoa	A tiny, round, quick-cooking seed grain with a visible internal ring. It comes in tan, red and black varietals. It naturally grows with a bitter-tasting saponin coating. Rinse before cooking.	Contains all essential amino acids, making it a complete protein. Source of fibre, phosphorus, magnesium, iron and folate.
Sesame	Tiny white or black seeds with a distinct nutty flavour. They are used to make tahini and toasted sesame oil.	Source of calcium, magnesium and iron. Excellent source of copper, an antioxidant.
Sunflower	Seeds from the centre of the beautiful yellow sunflower. Black-and-white striped outer seed coat opens to a grey elongated oval seed with terrific crunch.	Source of vitamin E, thiamin and the antioxidant selenium.

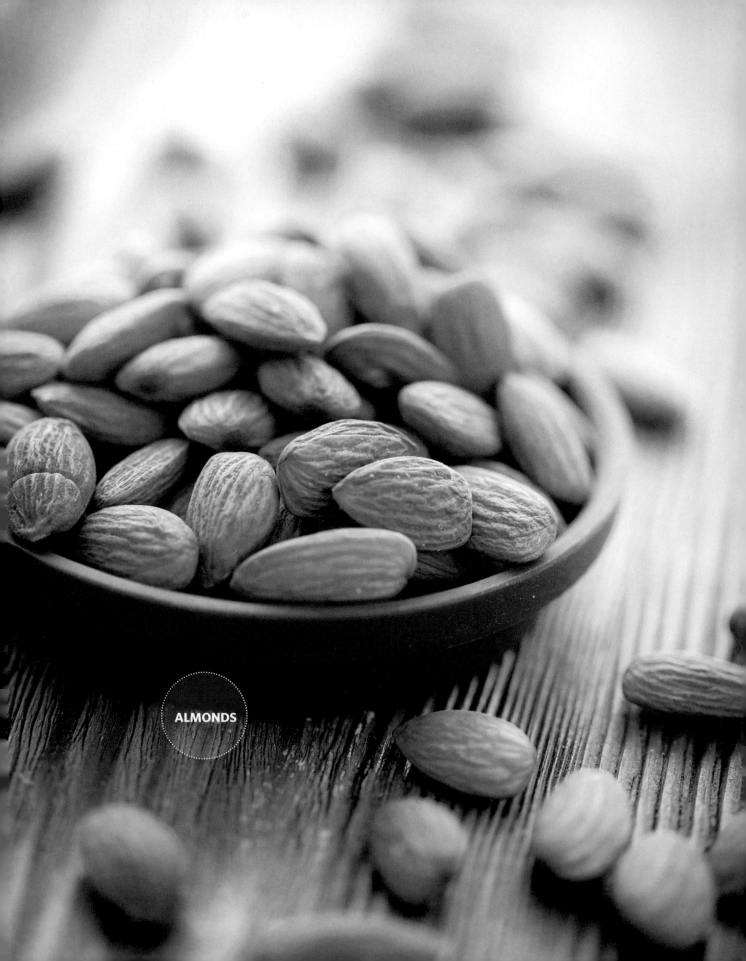

ALMONDS

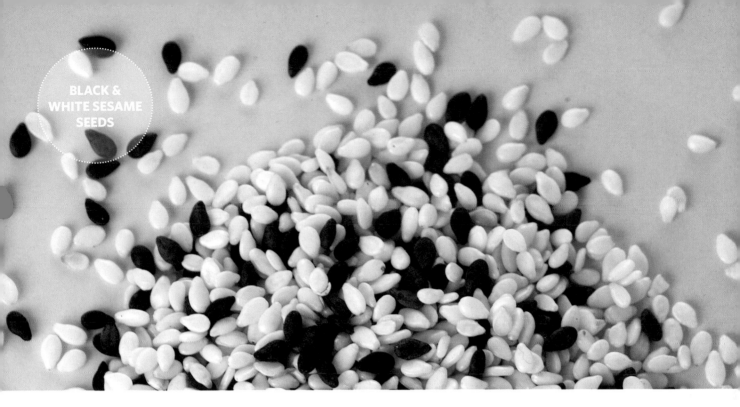

BLACK &
WHITE SESAME
SEEDS

TOASTING NUTS AND SEEDS

Toasting nuts and seeds intensifies their flavour and deepens their colour. It can be done in two ways:

In the oven

Preheat oven to 350°F (180°C). Line a rimmed baking sheet with parchment paper. Spread nuts or seeds out on the sheet and toast them in the middle of the oven until they are golden brown and aromatic, 8–12 minutes for nuts or 5–10 minutes for seeds, stirring once. Check every few minutes to ensure they do not burn. You can also toast nuts and seeds in a toaster oven, but since the heating elements are much closer to the nuts, they burn more easily, so watch them closely.

On the stovetop

In a cast iron skillet or frying pan, toast nuts or seeds over medium heat. Nuts take 5–6 minutes, seeds and small pine nuts about 3 minutes. Stir often. Watch them closely so they do not burn.

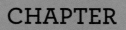

ORANGE GINGER FRUIT SALAD, P. 45

CHAPTER

3

Breakfast & Brunch

Tip: To serve, you can use this granola as part of trail mix, atop Greek yogurt, in parfaits, sprinkled on salad or as cereal with added milk.

Apricot Ginger Granola

My kids love Saturday mornings—it's the day we mix a batch of granola that will last the rest of the week. They like taking turns pouring, measuring and stirring their favourite grains, nuts, seeds and dried fruit, which we are able to switch up on a whim. This is a favoured combination of ours, thanks to the surprising warm spice of the candied ginger. Make sure to let the granola cool completely on the baking sheet; the ingredients adhere to each other as they cool, giving you those tell-tale clusters of true granola. —Cara

1. Preheat the oven to 325°F (160°C). Line a large rimmed baking sheet with parchment paper.

2. In a large bowl, stir together the oats, pistachios, pumpkin seeds, sesame seeds, sunflower seeds, cinnamon and cardamom.

3. In a small bowl, combine vanilla, olive oil and maple syrup. Stir to combine. Add to oat, nut and seed mixture.

4. Turn the mixture onto the baking sheet and spread in an even layer.

5. Bake until fragrant and golden brown, about 25–30 minutes.

6. Remove from the oven and let cool completely on the baking sheet.

7. Stir in the apricots and ginger once the granola is cool—about 20 minutes.

8. Store in an airtight container for 3–4 weeks.

MAKES 8 CUPS (2 L)

3 cups (750 mL) large flaked rolled oats

1 cup (250 mL) unsalted pistachios, chopped

1 cup (250 mL) raw unsalted pumpkin seeds

½ cup (125 mL) sesame seeds

½ cup (125 mL) raw unsalted sunflower seeds

¼ tsp (1 mL) ground cinnamon

½ tsp (2 mL) ground cardamom

½ tsp (2 mL) pure vanilla extract

½ cup (125 mL) extra virgin olive oil

½ cup (125 mL) pure maple syrup

½ cup (125 mL) finely chopped dried apricots

¼ cup (60 mL) chopped crystallized ginger

Tip: If you prefer a toned-down sweetness in your breakfast bowl, cut the maple syrup in this recipe to just ¼ cup (60 mL).

NUTRIENTS PER SERVING
SERVING SIZE: ¼ CUP (60 ML) GRANOLA

136 calories, 8 g fat, 1 g saturated fat, 2 mg sodium, 13 g carbohydrates, 2 g fibre, 5 g sugars, 4 g protein. Good source of magnesium.

Dried Cherry Almond Muesli

Growing up, I sat down to breakfast every morning with my dad, Jerry, the best role model for learning the importance of the morning meal. He never misses breakfast and has always told me it's the best way to start the day. And even though getting my kids ready for school leads to hectic mornings, we always make time for breakfast. I love muesli because you can mix it with yogurt the night before and refrigerate it overnight, shaving precious minutes off the morning routine. When the kids are at the breakfast table, I simply scoop the prepared muesli into bowls and we all enjoy breakfast together. Just like when I was growing up! —Cara

1. In a large bowl, combine the oats, bran, almonds, sunflower seeds, flaxseeds, cherries, salt and cinnamon.
2. Transfer to a large jar for storage for up to 3 months.

Tip: To prepare, scoop ½ cup (125 mL) muesli into ½ cup (125 mL) plain 2% Greek yogurt and mix to combine. Add berries if desired. Refrigerate overnight to allow muesli to soften. In the morning, remove the muesli from the fridge and enjoy with a drizzle of honey.

MAKES 6 CUPS (3 L)

3 cups (750 mL) large flaked rolled oats

¾ cup (175 mL) wheat bran or germ

¾ cup (175 mL) sliced raw almonds

¾ cup (175 mL) raw unsalted sunflower seeds

3 Tbsp (45 mL) ground flaxseeds

½ cup (125 mL) chopped dried cherries

¼ tsp (1 mL) sea salt

¼ tsp (1 mL) ground cinnamon

NUTRIENTS PER SERVING

SERVING SIZE: ½ CUP (125 mL) MUESLI, UNPREPARED

220 calories, 9 g fat, 1 g saturated fat, 50 mg sodium, 31 g carbohydrates, 7 g fibre, 6 g sugars, 7 g protein. Excellent source of magnesium. Good source of iron.

Fruity Oatmeal Pancakes

My kids adore these fruit-filled pancakes, which are perfect for a sleepy Sunday morning. The breakout flavour is the orange zest, so don't leave it out. I serve these with 2% Greek yogurt and a drizzle of pure maple syrup. Other soft fruit can replace the apples, kiwi or strawberries. —Cara

1. In a large bowl, combine the oats, buttermilk and orange juice. Set aside for 10 minutes.

2. Add the eggs and butter. Combine well.

3. Add flour, sugar, zest, baking powder, baking soda, cinnamon, nutmeg and salt; stir to mix well.

4. Gently fold in the fruit.

5. Heat a non-stick griddle over medium heat. Brush lightly with oil. Pour the batter in ¼ cupfuls (60 mL) onto the heated griddle. If batter seems runny, add another tablespoon of flour to thicken it.

6. Cook until golden-brown, about 4 minutes, then flip gently with a spatula. Cook the other side until golden brown, about 3 minutes.

7. Serve with optional toppings: a drizzle of pure maple syrup or honey, fresh fruit or Greek yogurt.

SERVES 8

2 cups (500 mL) large flaked rolled oats

1¾ cups (1 L) (410 mL) buttermilk

¼ cup (60 mL) orange juice

2 eggs, slightly beaten

¼ cup (60 mL) unsalted butter, melted

1 cup (250 mL) whole grain wheat or spelt flour

1 Tbsp (15 mL) sugar

2 tsp (10 mL) orange zest

1 tsp (5 mL) baking powder

1 tsp (5 mL) baking soda

¼ tsp (1 mL) ground cinnamon

Pinch of ground nutmeg

Pinch of sea salt

1 apple, peeled and finely diced

1 kiwi, peeled and finely diced

6 strawberries, finely diced

Olive oil, for grilling

Tip: If you don't have any buttermilk, you can make your own in minutes. Simply combine 1¾ cup (175 mL) milk with 1½ Tbsp (22 mL) lemon juice, stir and let it stand for 5–10 minutes. Voila—buttermilk!

NUTRIENTS PER SERVING SERVING SIZE: 2 PANCAKES

287 calories, 12 g fat, 5 g saturated fat, 289 mg sodium, 37 g carbohydrates, 5 g fibre, 7 g sugars, 10 g protein. Good source of thiamin and vitamin C.

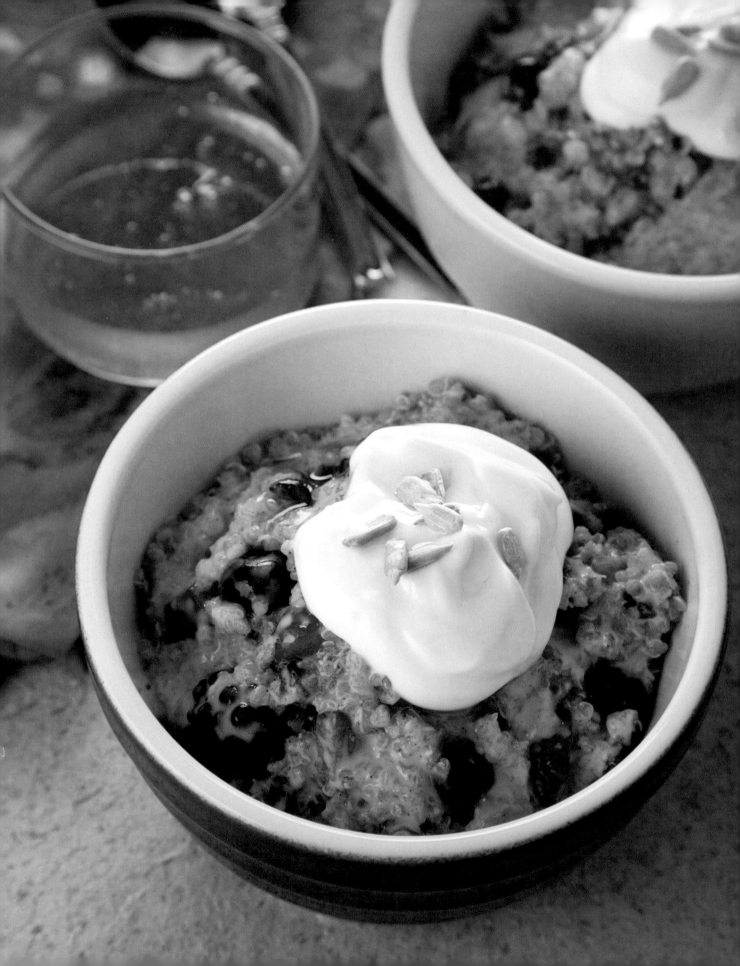

Quinoa & Berry Hot Cereal with Chai-Spiced Honey

This is a weekday staple at my house, and one of my eight-year-old daughter, Kasey's, favourite recipes. On my last birthday, this is what she made for my breakfast in bed! We use whatever fruit we have on-hand, as the results work equally well with any combination of berries. —Cara

1. In a large saucepan, combine the quinoa, milk, water, cinnamon and raisins. Cook over medium heat, stirring, until simmering. Cover, reduce heat to low and cook quinoa until most of the liquid is absorbed, about 15 minutes. Since it is a hot cereal reminiscent of porridge, it should still be somewhat runny and liquidy.

2. Stir in the maple syrup and berries. Let rest 5 for minutes.

3. Spoon into bowls and sprinkle with seeds.

4. Serve warm topped with Greek yogurt and Chai-Spiced Honey (optional).

Tip: If you are watching your sugar intake, you can prepare this using unsweetened soy beverage instead of milk, and omit the raisins. Those changes will bring the sugar content down to 7 grams per cup.

SERVES 4

1 cup (250 mL) quinoa, rinsed

2 cups (500 mL) skim milk or fortified soy beverage

1 cup (250 mL) water

1 tsp (5 mL) ground cinnamon

⅓ cup (75 mL) raisins

1 Tbsp (15 mL) pure maple syrup

2 cups (500 mL) mixed berries, fresh or frozen

⅓ cup (75 mL) unsalted sunflower seeds, toasted (see page 25)

1 cup (250 mL) 2% Greek yogurt (optional)

1 tsp (5 mL) Chai-Spiced Honey (see following page for recipe) (optional)

NUTRIENTS PER SERVING
SERVING SIZE: 1 CUP (250 ML) CEREAL

358 calories, 8 g fat, 1 g saturated fat, 72 mg sodium, 58 g carbohydrates, 7 g fibre, 20 g sugars, 13 g protein. Excellent source of riboflavin, folate, magnesium and zinc. Good source of thiamin, vitamin B_6, vitamin D, calcium and iron.

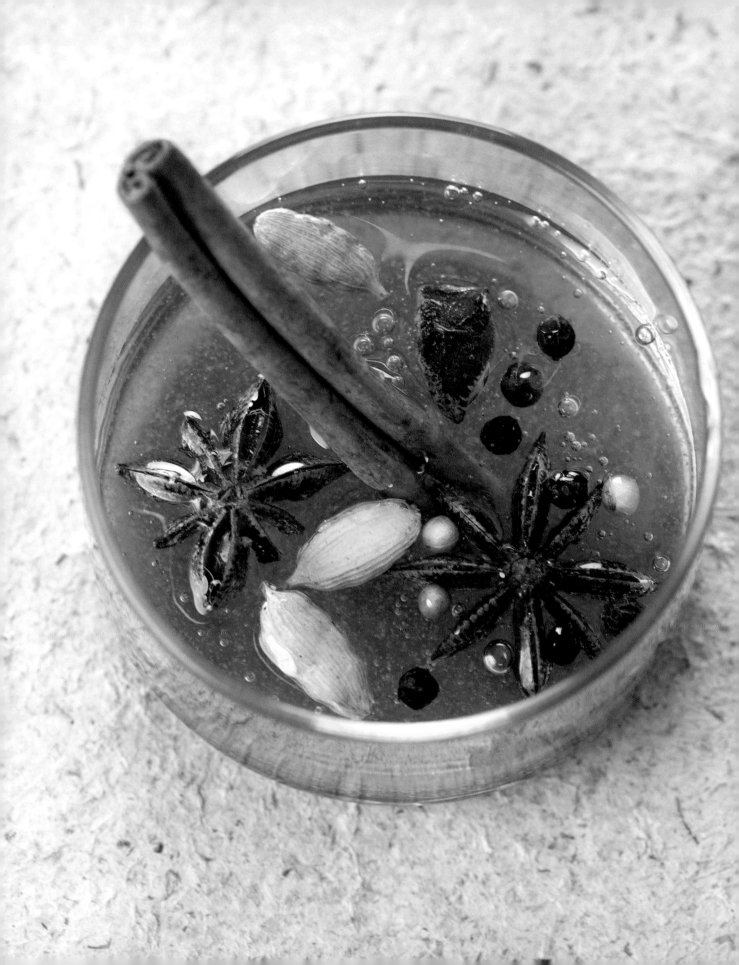

Chai-Spiced Honey

I love this spiced honey and the opportunity to use spice pods and sticks. Their fragrant scent and sturdiness make me feel at one with the earth. Only whole spices will work in this honey recipe! —Nettie

1. In a small saucepan over medium-low heat, warm honey. Add anise, cinnamon, cardamom, peppercorns and cloves.

2. Warm all ingredients together for 5 minutes. Don't let the honey come to a full boil. (If it boils, immediately reduce heat to low.)

3. Remove from heat and let the mixture sit in the saucepan for 20 minutes to let flavours infuse.

4. Once cool, use a fine-mesh sieve to strain the honey and remove solids.

5. Pour into a glass jar to store until ready to use. It will last 6 months. Do not refrigerate.

MAKES ½ CUP (125 ML)

½ cup (125 mL) honey

4 star anise pods

3 cinnamon sticks

3 cardamom pods

10 peppercorns

4 cloves

Tip: You can use this honey on yogurt, in oatmeal or stirred into warm milk or tea.

NUTRIENTS PER SERVING SERVING SIZE: 1 TSP (5 ML)
20 calories, 0 g fat, 0 g saturated fat, 0 mg sodium, 5 g carbohydrates, 0 g fibre, 5 g sugars, 0 g protein.

Frozen Fruit Smoothie

Smoothies are a family favourite, especially for my husband, Scott, and our four-year-old son, Aubrey. They love coming up with new concoctions using various fruits, and we always have frozen fruit on-hand for their experiments. Once a week, Scott powers up the blender (which he may like even more than the smoothie itself!) for a morning drink. When it's not this combination, it's something green—made with honeydew, kale and mint—to highlight Aubrey's favourite colour. —Cara

1. In a blender, add mango, raspberries, milk, yogurt, honey and hemp.
2. Cover and blend until smooth.
3. Pour into glasses and garnish with mint.
4. Serve immediately.

 Tip: If you are using frozen fruit, you do not need to add ice. If you are using fresh fruit, add 2 ice cubes.

SERVES 2 (OR 4 KID-SIZED PORTIONS)

1 cup (250 mL) frozen mango

1 cup (250 mL) frozen raspberries

1½ cups (500 mL) skim milk

½ cup (125 mL) 2% Greek yogurt

1 tsp (5 mL) honey

2 Tbsp (30 mL) hemp seeds

1 sprig fresh mint, for garnish

NUTRIENTS PER SERVING SERVING SIZE: ½ RECIPE

262 calories, 6 g fat, 1 g saturated fat, 120 mg sodium, 37 g carbohydrates, 6 g fibre, 29 g sugars, 16 g protein. Excellent source of vitamin A, riboflavin, vitamin B_{12}, vitamin C and vitamin D. Good source of calcium.

Quinoa Crunch Cereal

Breakfast cereal does not need to be high in sugar to be delicious. This crunchy combination is perfect on top of yogurt, or in a bowl with milk. We make this using high-quality, unrefined, organic canola oil from Quebec-based Maison Orphée, which has more flavour and a darker colour than regular canola oil. —Cara

1. Preheat the oven to 375°F (190°C). Line a rimmed baking sheet with parchment paper.
2. In a medium bowl, mix together quinoa, almonds, sesame seeds, maple syrup and oil. Spread on prepared baking sheet.
3. Bake until toasty and fragrant, 10–12 minutes.
4. Transfer to a bowl and let cool completely.
5. Store cereal in an airtight container at room temperature for up to 1 month. Serve atop yogurt or with milk.

MAKES 4 CUPS (1 L)

2 cups (500 mL) quinoa, rinsed

1 cup (250 mL) sliced raw almonds

¼ cup (60 mL) raw sesame seeds

2 Tbsp (30 mL) pure maple syrup

2 Tbsp (30 mL) organic canola oil

A Note About Milk

When cow's milk is not a dietary option, your next best bet to mimic its nutrient profile is fortified soy milk. It has the same amount of protein as cow's milk, and, has been enriched with copycat vitamins and minerals such as calcium and vitamin D. Milk alternatives such as almond, rice, oat, coconut or hemp milk do not contain a significant amount of protein (usually 1 gram vs 8–9 grams in cow's milk and soy milk). If you are looking for a protein-rich beverage, cow's milk or soy milk are your best choices.

NUTRIENTS PER SERVING

SERVING SIZE: ¼ CUP (60 ML) CEREAL

163 calories, 8 g fat, 1 g saturated fat, 2 mg sodium, 18 g carbohydrates, 3 g fibre, 2 g sugars, 5 g protein. Excellent source of magnesium. Good source of folate.

Tip: To serve, add ¼ cup (60 mL) to a small bowl with ½ cup (125 mL), milk or soy beverage. Allow ingredients to absorb milk for 5 minutes. Add fruit and enjoy.

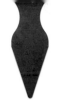

Crack-the-Code Breakfast Cereal

My 23-year-old bike-riding, scientist daughter Macko, eats this cereal every morning and swears she is not hungry until noon. She has experimented with the ingredients and finally uncovered the secret recipe to this delightful seed-based cereal, which sells for up to $15 per bag in the grocery store with names like Qi'a or Holy Crap. Visit a bulk store to buy raw ingredients and make your own—you'll save about 50 percent! —Nettie

1. In a medium bowl, combine chia, buckwheat, hemp seeds, cranberries, raisins, apple and cinnamon. Stir to combine.

 Tip: This serving size seems small, but chia seeds expand in liquid and take on a gelatinous, pudding-like consistency. If you prefer the visual cue of eating a fuller bowl of cereal, simply add our Crack-the-Code Breakfast Cereal to a whole grain puffed or flaked cereal and add milk or Greek yogurt.

MAKES 1¾ CUPS (425 ML)

¾ cup (175 mL) chia seeds

½ cup (125 mL) buckwheat groats

⅓ cup (75 mL) hemp seeds

1 Tbsp (15 mL) dried cranberries

1 Tbsp (15 mL) raisins

1 Tbsp (15 mL) finely chopped dried apple

½ tsp (2 mL) cinnamon

NUTRIENTS PER SERVING
SERVING SIZE: ¼ CUP (60 ML) CEREAL, UNPREPARED

184 calories, 10 g fat, 0 g saturated fat, 6 mg sodium, 20 g carbohydrates, 10 g fibre, 2 g sugars, 6 g protein.

Savoury Cheddar Scones

We used old cheddar cheese to give these scones a tangy bite. With firm cheeses such as cheddar, make sure to use a large (¼–½ inch/0.6–1 cm) teardrop shaped grater, rather than a small hand-held rasp grater with tiny holes—that way your shreds will be nice and thick. The shredding disk of a food processor can be used as well. When measuring, I always loosely pack a dry measuring cup for my grated cheese. As a time saver, you can always buy pre-grated cheese as well. Serve these alongside scrambled eggs and sliced tomatoes. —Nettie

1. Preheat oven to 375°F (190°C). Line a rimmed baking sheet with parchment paper.

2. In a large bowl, sift together the flour, baking powder, sugar and salt. Add cheddar and stir to mix well. Add the butter and rub into the flour mixture with your fingers until it resembles coarse cornmeal.

3. In a separate medium-sized bowl, whisk together the eggs and buttermilk for about 30 seconds. Pour the liquid over the flour mixture and stir until just combined.

4. Drop batter 1½ Tbsp (22 mL) at a time onto the prepared baking sheet to make 12 scones. Leave a 1-inch (2.5 cm) space in between for spreading.

5. Sprinkle each scone with pumpkin seeds.

6. Centring the cookie sheet on the middle oven rack, bake for 12–15 minutes, until the scones are golden brown and a tester inserted into the centre of each comes out clean.

7. Let cool on a wire rack. Enjoy.

MAKES 12 SCONES

1¾ cups (425 mL) whole grain spelt flour

2 tsp (10 mL) baking powder

1 Tbsp (15 mL) granulated sugar

½ tsp (2 mL) sea salt

¾ cup (175 mL) grated cheddar cheese

¼ cup (60 mL) unsalted butter

2 large eggs, lightly beaten

⅓ cup (75 mL) buttermilk

¼ cup (60 mL) unsalted pumpkin seeds, toasted (see page 25)

A Note About Spelt

Spelt is a relative to wheat, and can be used in place of wheat flour in cooking and baking. When buying it, look for stone-ground 100% whole grain spelt flour. If it doesn't say "whole grain," it has likely been refined, which removes the fibre and most of the vitamins and minerals, making it less nutritious. Since spelt is in the wheat family, it is not a gluten-free grain.

NUTRIENTS PER SERVING
SERVING SIZE: 1 SCONE

168 calories, 10 g fat, 5 g saturated fat, 235 mg sodium, 13 g carbohydrates, 2 g fibre, 1 g sugars, 6 g protein.

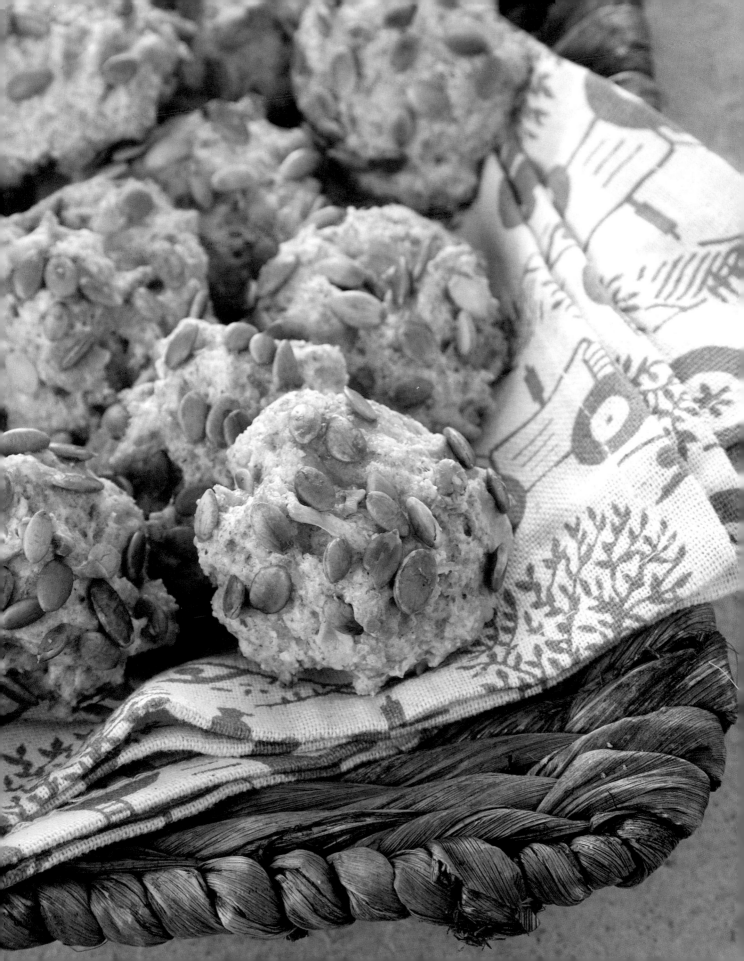

Black Bean Breakfast Burritos

When I go away to my cottage on Ontario's Bella Lake, I leave my husband, Jim, two dozen black bean burritos to eat morning, noon or night. They freeze so well! You can let them thaw overnight in the refrigerator or thaw in the microwave and heat-to-eat. Use a spicy salsa for an extra-bold flavour. —Nettie

1. In a heavy skillet, heat 2 tsp (10 mL) oil over medium heat. Sauté the onion and potato for 5 minutes, until soft and starting to turn golden.

2. Add the beans, salsa and chili powder to the skillet and cook for 3–5 minutes, slightly mashing some of the beans with a fork, until heated through. Transfer the mixture to a bowl.

3. In a medium-sized bowl, whisk together the eggs.

4. Heat remaining 1 tsp (5 mL) oil in the skillet. Add the eggs. Stir the eggs around with a spatula to scramble them. Once scrambled, combine with the bean mixture.

5. Divide one-quarter of the egg and bean mixture among the four tortillas, spreading it down the middle and leaving space on the sides and at both ends. Top with cheese, avocado and fresh cilantro (if using).

6. Fold over one long side to cover the filling, fold over both short ends, then roll the whole thing over to close up into a package.

7. Serve warm, with cilantro, extra salsa and sour cream, if desired.

Tip: Most of our recipes that use canned beans recommend the two-step "drain and rinse" process. This is usually to rinse the salt and canning liquid off the beans. Our recipes use no-salt-added beans, so we rinse only to remove the mush-like cooking liquid. In this recipe, beans are not rinsed! Since the black beans are mashed, the canning liquid helps by adding moisture to the beans and it's smart to leave it in.

MAKES 4 BURRITOS

1 Tbsp (15 mL) extra virgin olive oil, divided

1 onion, finely diced

1 medium red potato, coarsely grated

14 oz (400 g) can no-salt-added black beans, drained

½ cup (125 mL) salsa

2 tsp (10 mL) chili powder

4 large eggs

4 whole grain tortillas (10 inches/25 cm each)

½ cup (125 mL) shredded cheddar or Monterey Jack cheese

1 ripe avocado, sliced

¼ cup (60 mL) chopped fresh cilantro, for garnish (optional)

Sour cream and extra salsa, for serving (optional)

NUTRIENTS PER SERVING
SERVING SIZE: 1 BURRITO

527 calories, 23 g fat, 7 g saturated fat, 760 mg sodium, 58 g carbohydrates, 14 g fibre, 6 g sugars, 23 g protein. Excellent source of folate and vitamin B_{12}. Good source of riboflavin, vitamin B_6, calcium, iron and zinc.

Scrambled Eggs with Black Beans & Salsa

The jalapeno pepper really enhances this recipe. A popular, mid-range spicy pepper, jalapenos can be found in both green and red. I always wear thin rubber gloves when slicing chilies due to the presence of their volatile oils that can cause discomfort if you touch your mouth or eyes after cutting them bare-handed. Black beans, eggs and salsa are a most satisfying meal because you have lots of flavour and a colourful plate. —Nettie

1. In a small bowl, combine cilantro, tomatoes, red peppers, onion, jalapeno and lime juice. Toss to combine. Cover and refrigerate until ready to use.

2. In a medium non-stick pan over medium heat, heat 1 Tbsp (15 mL) of oil. Sauté mushrooms, onions and peppers in the pan until soft, about 5 minutes. Add the beans and cook for 2 more minutes. Remove from the heat. Put bean mixture into a bowl.

3. In a small bowl, whisk the eggs, salt and milk together.

4. In the same non-stick pan, heat the remaining tablespoon of oil over medium heat. Add the egg mixture and scramble until no longer runny.

5. Add the bean mixture back into the non-stick pan and cook everything together for 2–3 minutes, stirring with a wooden spoon or spatula. Remove from the heat and cover to keep warm.

6. Serve eggs immediately topped with salsa.

SERVES 6

Salsa

½ cup (125 mL) chopped fresh cilantro

1 large tomato, diced

½ red pepper, diced

¼ red onion, diced

1 small jalapeno pepper, seeded and minced

2 Tbsp (30 mL) fresh lime juice

Eggs

2 Tbsp (30 mL) olive oil, divided

½ cup (125 mL) sliced shiitake mushrooms

4 sliced green onions

1 yellow pepper, diced

14 oz (410 mL) can no-salt-added black beans

6 large eggs

1 tsp (5 mL) sea salt

¼ cup (60 mL) 2% milk

Tip: Cilantro is sometimes called coriander when you buy the fresh herb, but usually coriander refers to the dried seed or ground spice, and cilantro refers to the fresh leafy herbs. They are all part of the same plant.

NUTRIENTS PER SERVING SERVING SIZE: ⅙ RECIPE

307 calories, 12 g fat, 2 g saturated fat, 700 mg sodium, 37 g carbohydrates, 6 g fibre, 5 g sugars, 15 g protein. Very high in fibre. Excellent source of riboflavin, folate, vitamin B12, vitamin C, magnesium, iron and zinc. Good source of vitamin A, thiamin and niacin.

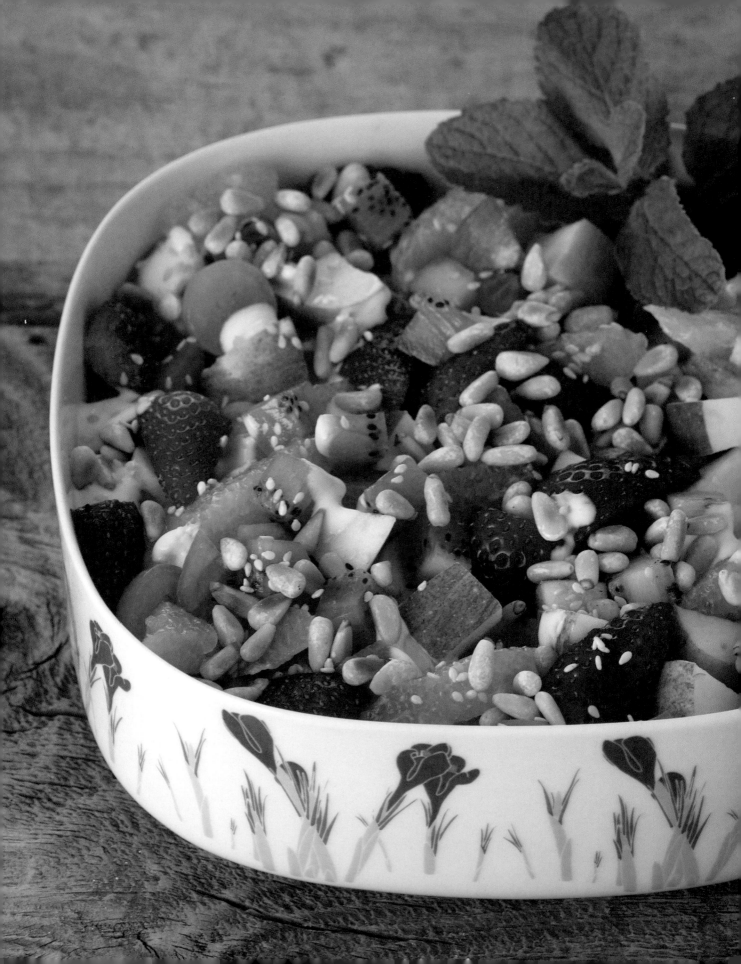

Orange Ginger Fruit Salad

Nothing makes me happier than eating a fresh fruit salad, especially after a refreshing swim in Ontario's Bella Lake with my friends Kathy and Barbara. They adore crystallized ginger and adding it to fruit salad. While ginger is usually spicy, crystallized ginger is sweet—it is made by cooking sliced pieces of fresh ginger in heavy sugar syrup, replacing all moisture with the sugar. The ginger is then coated with more sugar and dried. It can give unripe fruit a boost of needed sweetness. —Nettie

1. In a medium bowl, add strawberries, grapes, apple, orange and kiwi.

2. In a small bowl, whisk the orange juice, yogurt, ginger and honey. Pour the dressing over the fruit. Cover and refrigerate for a few hours to marry the flavours.

3. Serve and garnishing with pine nuts, sesame seeds and mint.

A Note About Greek Yogurt

With double the protein and half the carbohydrate content of regular yogurt, double-strained Greek yogurt was a staple ingredient in this book. It's so rich and creamy that we even used it as a substitute for sour cream in most of our recipes. If you prefer fat-free or 1% yogurt, feel free to use that as a substitute for 2%—it doesn't change the high protein content. Greek yogurts with 8–10% fat are not really necessary, since the lower-fat versions are already decadently thick and creamy.

MAKES 10 SERVINGS

2 cups (500 mL) hulled and sliced strawberries

2 cups (500 mL) grapes

2 unpeeled apples, diced

3 oranges, peeled and cubed

2 kiwi, peeled and diced

¼ cup (60 mL) orange juice

1 cup (250 mL) 2% Greek yogurt

¼ cup (60 mL) chopped crystallized ginger

1 Tbsp (15 mL) honey

2 Tbsp (30 mL) pine nuts, toasted

2 Tbsp (30 mL) sesame seeds, toasted

⅓ cup (75 mL) chopped fresh mint leaves

NUTRIENTS PER SERVING
SERVING SIZE: 1 CUP (250 ML) SALAD

110 calories, 2 g fat, 0 g saturated fat, 11 mg sodium, 21 g carbohydrates, 3 g fibre, 14 g sugars, 3 g protein. Excellent source of vitamin C.

Spicy Brunch Home Fries

If you like spice, these are the potatoes for you! These are the spiciest potatoes I prepare, and if you do not have the three types of chili powder required in the recipe, you can easily substitute with what you have on-hand. I especially like combining ancho and chipotle chili powders, as the flavour is well rounded and just hot enough for my taste buds. —Nettie

1. Preheat the oven to 400°F (200°C).
2. In a medium-sized bowl, toss potatoes with oil, salt and chili powders.
3. Line a rimmed baking sheet with parchment paper. Spread potatoes onto baking sheet.
4. Roast for 30 minutes, or until golden brown on the outside and soft in the middle. Stir potatoes halfway through roasting.
5. Add roasted potatoes to a large serving bowl. Add garam masala, salt and pepper. Serve hot.

 Tip: Don't refrigerate your spuds. Cold temperatures convert potatoes' starch to sugar, resulting in a sweet taste and discolouration when cooked.

SERVES 6

4 medium red potatoes, diced to 1-inch (2.5 cm) squares

2 Tbsp (30 mL) extra virgin olive oil

½ tsp (2 mL) sea salt

½ tsp (2 mL) ground ancho chili powder

¼ tsp (1 mL) cayenne chili powder

¼ tsp (1 mL) ground chipotle chili powder

1 tsp (5 mL) garam masala

¼ tsp (1 mL) sea salt

¼ tsp (1 mL) freshly ground black pepper

NUTRIENTS PER SERVING
SERVING SIZE: ⅙ RECIPE

207 calories, 8 g fat, 1 g saturated fat, 223 mg sodium, 30 g carbohydrates, 4 g fibre, 4 g sugars, 4 g protein. Excellent source of vitamin A. Good source of folate, vitamin C and magnesium.

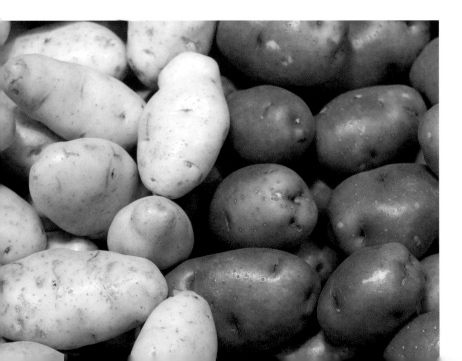

Scrambled Tofu

I have been eating tofu for over 40 years. The variety and packaging keeps getting better and better. No more leaky tubs of tofu, and what a choice in texture! When Cameron and Macko were little kids, this recipe was their version of scrambled eggs. They believed I had added eggs to the tofu because the turmeric coloured the tofu a bright yellow. These do look like scrambled eggs—but may taste even better. —Nettie

1. Drain the tofu and crumble it into a small bowl.
2. In a medium sauté pan on medium heat, add olive oil. Sauté the garlic and peppers for about 2 minutes.
3. Stir in the tofu.
4. Add turmeric, salt, pepper, green onions, peas, spinach and tamari.
5. Cook the tofu for 3 more minutes, stirring occasionally.
6. Garnish with basil and sesame seeds.
7. Serve as is or, optionally, serve with whole grain toast.

SERVES 6

12 oz (350 g) organic firm tofu

2 Tbsp (30 mL) extra virgin olive oil

1 garlic clove, sliced thin

¼ red pepper, diced

½ tsp (2 mL) turmeric

½ tsp (2 mL) sea salt

¼ tsp (1 mL) freshly ground black pepper

6 sliced green onions

½ cup (125 mL) peas, fresh or frozen

2 cups (500 mL) baby spinach leaves, washed

2 tsp (10 mL) sodium-reduced tamari

½ cup (125 mL) chopped fresh basil, for garnish

2 Tbsp (30 mL) sesame seeds, toasted (see page 25), for garnish

A Note About Turmeric

Turmeric, which is part of the ginger family, has a peppery, warm, bitter flavour. It's a well-known ingredient in curry powder and is often used to add a bright yellow colour to recipes. The root of turmeric is also used widely to make medicine; it's been researched as a treatment for its use as an anti-inflammatory and may help with arthritis, heartburn, digestive disorders and depression. It's important to note that the therapeutic dose of certain spices for treatment of health conditions is more than the sprinkle used in most recipes.

NUTRIENTS PER SERVING SERVING SIZE: ⅙ RECIPE

166 calories, 11 g fat, 2 g saturated fat, 311 mg sodium, 6 g carbohydrates, 2 g fibre, 1 g sugars, 11 g protein. Good source of iron.

Tip: Savoury yogurt is so trendy right now! So, we made a little extra for you to keep in the fridge. You can use it as a dip for crackers or vegetables, a sauce for fish, or add cucumbers and olives and enjoy it as is, right out of the bowl. That's how it's served at Sohha, a savoury yogurt stand in New York City's Chelsea Market.

Broccoli Brunch Patties

Dear Reader, I'm not a fan of ordinary pancakes, and I don't really like maple syrup either. That's why I'm so glad that we developed this delicious savoury pancake, complete with a yogurt dipping sauce. It's an excellent addition to any brunch table, and they freeze well too. —Nettie

1. Set a collapsible steamer basket in a large pot. Add enough water to reach the bottom of the steamer basket. Bring to a boil over high heat. Place the broccoli in the steamer basket, cover and steam for 3–5 minutes, or until tender. Set aside.

2. Place ground flax in a small bowl. Add water. Stir well. Allow to stand for 3 minutes.

3. Put the steamed broccoli, onion, chili and garlic in a food processor and pulse on and off to coarsely chop (do not purée the vegetables), or chop by hand.

4. Transfer the chopped ingredients to a large mixing bowl and stir in the oil, flour, dill and salt. Add the ground flax mixture, egg, milk and paprika. Mix thoroughly with a wooden spoon.

5. In non-stick skillet, heat 1 tsp (5 mL) of butter over medium heat. Using ¼ cup (60 mL) batter for each pancake, add three ¼ cup (60 mL) amounts in a frying pan large enough to allow the patties to be far enough apart so that they don't touch.

6. Cook over medium heat for 3–4 minutes. Flip patties and cook the other side for 3 minutes. Transfer them to a hot platter to keep warm. Add 1 tsp (5 mL) of butter to the skillet for each new batch.

7. To serve, mix all of the ingredients for the yogurt dip together and spoon 1 tsp (5 mL) on top of each pancake.

NUTRIENTS PER SERVING
SERVING SIZE: 2 PATTIES WITH 2 TSP (10 ML) YOGURT

256 calories, 16 g fat, 4 g saturated fat, 150 mg sodium, 22 g carbohydrates, 3 g fibre, 3 g sugars, 7 g protein. Excellent source of folate and vitamin D.

SERVES 6

4 cups (1 L) broccoli florets

1 Tbsp (15 mL) flaxseeds, finely ground

3 Tbsp (45 mL) water

1 onion, diced

1 small hot chili pepper, seeded and diced, or ½ tsp (2 mL) chili powder

2 garlic cloves, minced

¼ cup (60 mL) extra virgin olive oil

⅔ cup (150 mL) whole grain wheat flour

1 Tbsp (15 mL) finely chopped fresh dill

¼ tsp (1 mL) sea salt

1 large egg

⅓ cup (75 mL) 2% milk

1 tsp (5 mL) smoked paprika

4 tsp (20 mL) unsalted butter, divided

Yogurt dipping sauce

1 cup (250 mL) plain 2% Greek yogurt

1 Tbsp (15 mL) fresh lemon juice

½ tsp (2 mL) hot sauce

⅛ tsp (0.5 mL) sea salt

⅛ tsp (0.5 mL) freshly ground black pepper

Sprinkling of chopped fresh dill

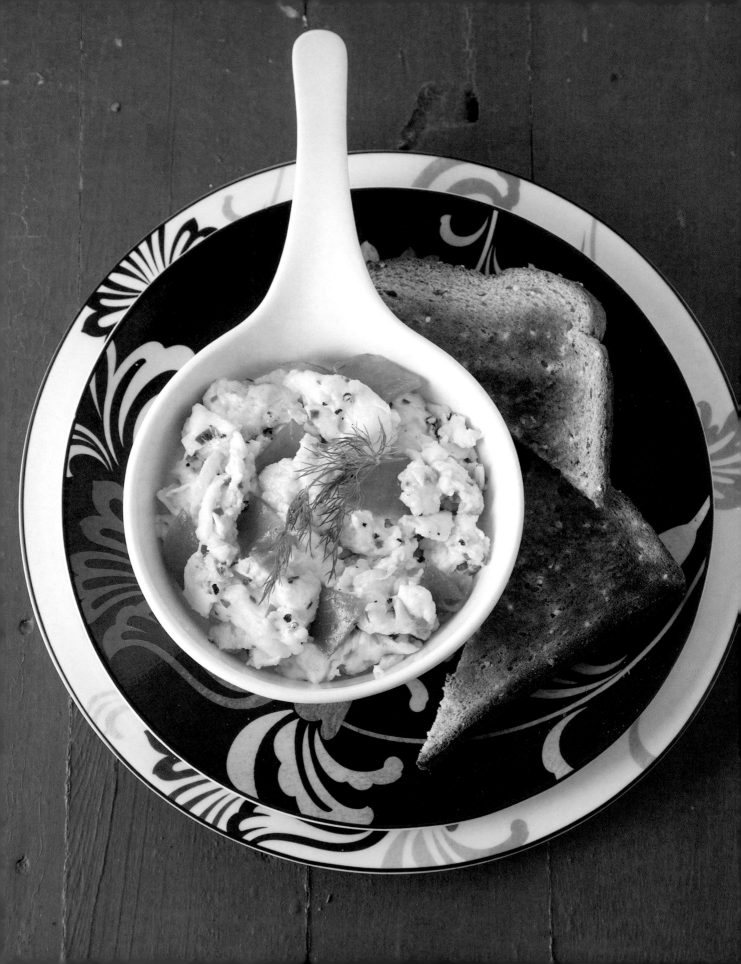

Smoked Salmon Scramble

Skip the bagel and cream cheese and use lox in your eggs instead! Smoked salmon is so rich and flavourful that a little bit goes a long way in this elegant take on scrambled eggs. This delicious combination is accented by fresh dill and toasted sesame seeds, and it is best served with whole grain toast. You can also add a few capers as the final garnish. —Cara

1. In a small bowl, whisk together eggs, milk and salt. Set aside.
2. Heat a non-stick skillet over medium heat. Add butter. Once butter has melted, add green onions; sauté for 1 minute.
3. Add the egg mix and gently scramble until the eggs are set.
4. Add in smoked salmon for the last minute of cooking the eggs.
5. Divide among 4 plates and top with dill and sesame seeds.
6. Serve with toasted flax bread.

A Note About Sesame Seeds

Black sesame seeds are not hulled, while white sesame seeds are stripped of their hull. But this doesn't mean that white sesame seeds are just black ones with no shells! In fact, they are two different varieties from the same flowering sesame plant. One major difference is that the black seeds are higher in calcium, which is found in the hulls. Black sesame seeds add a wonderful hit of surprising colour; they have a nutty, smoky flavour and a crispier texture than white seeds, which are sweeter. Because they are quite different, they're terrific when used in combination.

SERVES 4

8 eggs

¼ cup (60 mL) skim milk

¼ tsp (1 mL) sea salt

1 Tbsp (15 mL) unsalted butter

2 green onions, minced

2 oz (60 g) smoked salmon lox, cut into bite-sized pieces

2 Tbsp (30 mL) chopped fresh dill

1 Tbsp (15 mL) toasted sesame seeds (see page 25)

4 slices whole grain flax bread

NUTRIENTS PER SERVING
SERVING SIZE: ¼ RECIPE

344 calories, 18 g fat, 6 g saturated fat, 588 mg sodium, 24 g carbohydrates, 3 g fibre, 5 g sugars, 21 g protein. Excellent source of riboflavin, folate, vitamin D, vitamin B$_{12}$, magnesium and zinc. Good source of vitamin A, thiamin and iron.

Amaranth Millet Porridge with Pistachio Seed Sprinkle

Amaranth and millet are well-suited for making porridge since they both become slightly sticky and oatmeal-like when cooked with liquid. Simmering these whole grains in milk or soy beverage instead of water will add more protein, vitamins and minerals to this breakfast meal. Extra porridge can be refrigerated and reheated the next morning with a few extra tablespoons of milk. —Cara

1. Preheat oven to 350°F (180°C). Line a rimmed baking sheet with parchment paper.

2. Put pistachios, pumpkin seeds, sunflower seeds, hemp seeds, sesame seeds and sugar in a small bowl and stir to combine. Spread mixture over baking sheet and bake for 8–10 minutes or until golden. Set aside to cool.

3. In a medium-sized pot, combine millet, amaranth and cinnamon with water and 1 cup (250 mL) of milk and bring to a boil. Reduce heat to low, cover and simmer, stirring occasionally, about 20 minutes or until water is absorbed.

4. Add the remaining 1 cup (250 mL) milk and apple, cover and simmer, stirring occasionally for 10 minutes or until porridge is thick and creamy and the grains are tender.

5. Serve the porridge topped with ¼ cup (60 mL) Greek yogurt, and 2 Tbsp (30 mL) of the seed sprinkle. Top with ½ tsp (2 mL) of honey (if using).

Tip: The leftover seed sprinkle can be enjoyed as a snack, used on Greek yogurt or saved for tomorrow's porridge.

SERVES 4

Pistachio seed sprinkle

¼ cup (60 mL) unsalted pistachios, chopped

¼ cup (60 mL) raw unsalted pumpkin seeds

¼ cup (60 mL) raw unsalted sunflower seeds

¼ cup (60 mL) hemp seeds

¼ cup (60 mL) sesame seeds

1½ Tbsp (22 mL) light brown sugar

Porridge

¾ cup (175 mL) millet

¼ cup (60 mL) amaranth

1 tsp (5 mL) ground cinnamon

2 cups (500 mL) water

2 cups (500 mL) 1% milk or fortified soy beverage, divided

1 medium unpeeled apple, shredded

1 cup (250 mL) 2% plain Greek yogurt, to serve

2 tsp (10 mL) honey, to serve (optional)

NUTRIENTS PER SERVING SERVING SIZE: 1 CUP (250 ML) PORRIDGE WITH ¼ CUP (60 ML) YOGURT AND 2 TBSP (30 ML) SPRINKLE

427 calories, 13 g fat, 3 g saturated fat, 59 mg sodium, 63 g carbohydrates, 8 g fibre, 14 g sugars, 18 g protein. Excellent source of folate, magnesium and iron. Good source of thiamin, vitamin B_6, calcium and zinc.

Red Buckwheat Hash

You can buy buckwheat groats, which are often called kasha, in the rice section or kosher section of most grocery stores. Read the box carefully when you buy it to ensure you are getting whole groats, since buckwheat also comes in coarse, medium and fine granulation (buckwheat flour). —Nettie

SERVES 6

2 medium sweet potatoes, peeled and diced

3 small red beets, peeled and diced

¼ cup (60 mL) chopped fresh dill

14 oz (410 mL) can no-salt-added cannellini beans, drained

½ tsp (2 mL) sea salt, divided

½ tsp (2 mL) freshly ground pepper, divided

2 Tbsp (30 mL) extra virgin olive oil

1 Vidalia or other sweet onion, diced

3 garlic cloves, minced

1 large egg

1 cup (250 mL) buckwheat groats

1½ cups (500 mL) boiling water

¾ cup (175 mL) crumbled feta cheese

¼ cup (60 mL) plain 2% Greek yogurt

2 Tbsp (30 mL) chopped fresh chives, for serving

1. In a large bowl, stir together sweet potatoes, beets, dill, beans, ¼ tsp (1 mL) salt and ¼ tsp (1 mL) pepper. Set aside.

2. In a large non-stick saucepan, heat olive oil over medium heat. Add onion and sauté until soft and translucent, about 4 minutes. Add garlic and cook for 1 minute.

3. Pour the sweet potato and bean mixture into the saucepan and stir to combine with onions. Stir so it forms an even layer in the pan. Use a spatula to press down the layer so it's flat. Cover and cook until the potatoes are fork-tender, about 30 minutes, flipping after 15 minutes so both sides brown evenly. After flipping, press mixture down again. It can fall apart a bit, but it's a rustic hash, so that's okay!

4. Lightly beat egg in a bowl. Add buckwheat groats and stir until well coated. Heat a saucepan over medium heat. Add buckwheat and toast, stirring constantly for 3 minutes or until the grains begin to separate and are fragrant.

5. Add boiling water, and remaining salt and pepper. Cover, reduce heat and simmer for 8–10 minutes, or until most of the water is absorbed. Remove from heat and let stand without lid for 5 minutes.

6. Once beets and potatoes are fork-tender, stir in the cooked buckwheat groats.

7. Transfer cooked saucepan ingredients to a large bowl. Add feta. Mix well.

8. To serve, scoop into 6 individual bowls and dollop with Greek yogurt and chives.

NUTRIENTS PER SERVING SERVING SIZE: ⅙ RECIPE

318 calories, 11 g fat, 4 g saturated fat, 541 mg sodium, 46 g carbohydrates, 8 g fibre, 11 g sugars, 12 g protein. Very high in fibre. Excellent source of vitamin A, thiamin, vitamin B_6, folate and magnesium. Good source of riboflavin, vitamin B_{12}, calcium, iron and zinc.

Breakfast Eggs & Beans

Favas are large oval beans, golden brown when dried and green when fresh. Nutty and creamy in texture, they are ready to use when purchased canned. Oh, the convenience! Fresh fava beans are available in spring. They need to be shucked from their bulky green pod and after blanching, removed from their tough outer skin. Substitute lima beans or edamame if favas are unavailable. —Nettie

1. In small-sized non-stick pan over medium heat, toast cumin until fragrant, about 1 minute.

2. In a medium-sized saucepan, heat oil over medium heat. Add garlic and red onions. Sauté at medium heat for 3–5 minutes, stirring often. Add cumin and fava beans. Lower heat to a simmer and cook for 10 minutes. Mash the beans with a fork.

3. Add dill and tomatoes. Cook for 5 more minutes.

4. Spoon the beans into 4 portions and garnish each with an egg. Sprinkle with salt and pepper.

5. Serve immediately, garnishing with lemon wedges.

Tip: You may have noticed that all of the recipes in the book recommend using beans with no added salt, except for this one. Why? We could not find any brand of canned fava beans that are made without salt! It's not a concern though. If you use a sieve or strainer to drain and rinse your canned fava beans, you will eliminate about 40 percent of the sodium.

SERVES 4

2 tsp (10 mL) ground cumin

¼ cup (60 mL) extra virgin olive oil

4 garlic cloves, minced

½ red onion, diced

19 oz (560 mL) can fava beans, drained and rinsed

2 Tbsp (30 mL) finely chopped fresh dill

3 small ripe tomatoes (such as plum tomatoes), quartered

4 hard-boiled eggs, sliced into quarters

¼ tsp (1 mL) sea salt

⅛ tsp (0.5 mL) freshly ground black pepper

1 lemon, sliced into wedges

NUTRIENTS PER SERVING SERVING SIZE: ¼ RECIPE

313 calories, 20 g fat, 4 g saturated fat, 220 mg sodium, 23 g carbohydrates, 6 g fibre, 4 g sugars, 13 g protein. Excellent source of folate. Good source of riboflavin, magnesium, iron and zinc.

A Note About Breakfast

If you are starting your day with a donut or toaster pastry, you're not giving your body the fuel it needs for optimal performance. A sugar rush provides are quick burst of power, but no sustained energy. For a morning filled with better concentration and no rumbling stomach, a balanced breakfast should contain:

- Fibre, to help you feel full for longer
- Some carbohydrate, for immediate energy
- Protein for sustained energy
- A source of healthy fat, to slow digestion
- Fluid, for healthy hydration

Fibre and carbohydrates come from whole grains, fruit, nuts and legumes. Your best protein choices include eggs, nuts, seeds, nut butter, Greek yogurt, milk, fortified soy beverage and cheese. All of our breakfast recipes are built on these components!

Research shows that people who eat breakfast:

- Have better concentration and alertness, whether in the classroom or the boardroom
- Have more strength and endurance when engaging in physical activity
- Are better able to manage their weight
- Get more nutrients throughout the day and have higher intakes of fibre, vitamins and minerals compared to those who skip breakfast

After a night of fasting while asleep, our bodies need a boost of energy to function effectively and efficiently in the morning. It's important to make time for a healthy breakfast every day.

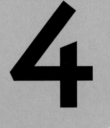

CHAPTER
4

Appetizers

Tip: While red beets are the most common to find, you can also buy golden beets and striped "candy cane" beets at some grocery stores. All types will work well in this recipe; sometimes I use all three to add spectacular colour.

Beets with Spicy Goat Cheese & Pumpkin Seed Pralines

Every year in April, I invite my friend James over for dinner when the rest of his family travels during Passover. Since he observes the holiday, I serve a menu without leavened bread, which means no topped baguette slices for appetizers. To please his palate, one year I asked him to describe the flavours he enjoys the most and came up with this custom-made *amuse-bouche*. He loved it, and it turns out that everyone else loved it too; it has become a dinner party staple ever since. —Cara

1. Place beets in a large pot and cover with water. Bring to a rolling boil and cook until fork-tender, about 1 hour. Let cool, peel and slice into ¼-inch (6 mm) thick rounds. Arrange on a large platter.

2. Bring a small pan to medium heat, and add sugar and pumpkin seeds. Stir until sugar liquefies and coats the seeds, about 8 minutes. Continue to stir for 1–2 minutes, being careful not to let them burn. Set aside to cool.

3. In a bowl, mix softened goat cheese with the cayenne, salt and pepper.

4. To assemble, place beets on a large platter. Top each beet round with a dot of balsamic glaze, ½ tsp (2 mL) of goat cheese and a small cluster of pumpkin seed pralines.

SERVES 10

8 medium beets

1 Tbsp (15 mL) granulated sugar

¼ cup (60 mL) raw unsalted pumpkin seeds

4.5 oz (130 g) package goat cheese, softened at room temperature for 10 minutes

¼ tsp (1 mL) cayenne pepper

⅛ tsp (0.5 mL) kosher salt

⅛ tsp (0.5 mL) freshly ground black pepper

1 Tbsp (15 mL) balsamic glaze

Tip: Balsamic glaze is a thick, sweet, syrupy version of balsamic vinegar that's found in the oil and vinegar section of the grocery store. Depending on the brand you buy, it may be called balsamic glaze, balsamic syrup or balsamic reduction.

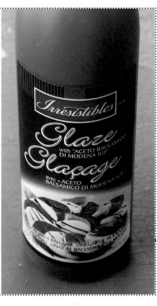

NUTRIENTS PER SERVING
SERVING SIZE: 4 ROUNDS

96 calories, 6 g fat, 2 g saturated fat, 120 mg sodium, 8 g carbohydrates, 2 g fibre, 6 g sugars, 4 g protein.

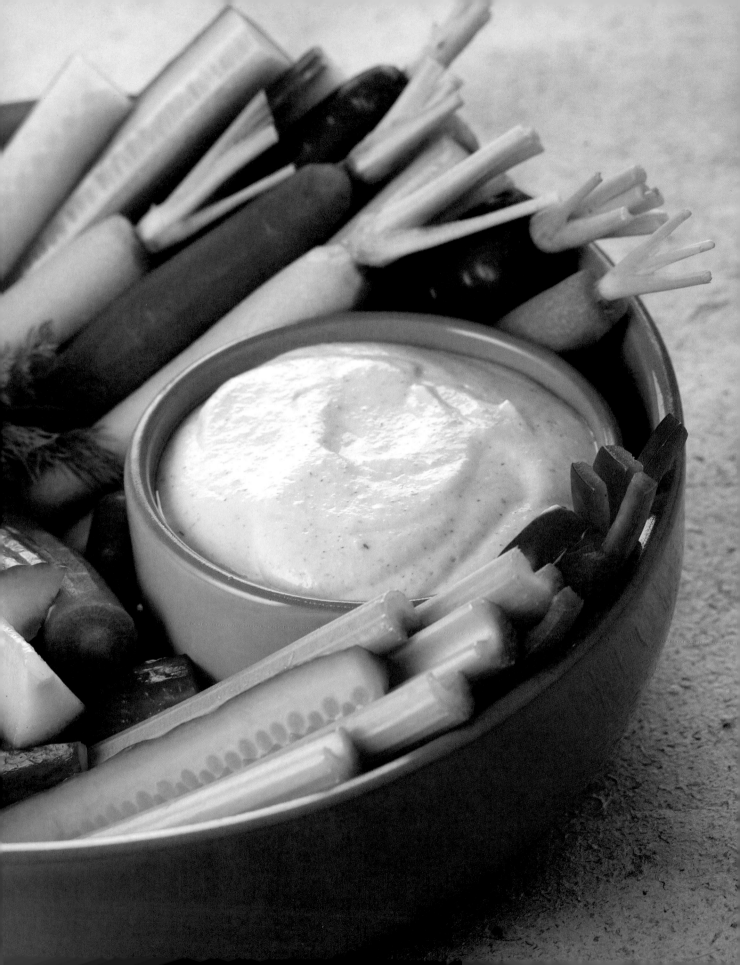

Green Goddess Dip

I often tell parents that using dip is a great way to entice their children to eat more vegetables—most kids like the fun of dunking and the mess of dipping! Commercial dips and processed salad dressings may be high in salt, fat and sugar. Instead of using those, I whip up this healthier ranch-like Green Goddess dip, which takes about five minutes, and can last about five days in the fridge. Though in my house, it's usually gone by day two! It also makes a lovely sauce for baked salmon or sea bass. —Cara

1. In a food processor, combine all ingredients. Process for about 1 minute or until puréed.
2. Pair this dip with fresh vegetables such as carrot, jicama, red pepper, celery, grape tomatoes and cucumber.

 Tip: Be picky about your pickles. Some brands needlessly use artificial colours and flavours, and a host of preservatives. Look for a clean ingredient list with little more than cucumber, vinegar, garlic, dill (or other herbs and spices) and salt.

NUTRIENTS PER SERVING
SERVING SIZE: 2 TBSP (30 ML) DIP

47 calories, 4 g fat, 0 g saturated fat, 108 mg sodium, 2 g carbohydrates, 0 g fibre, 1 g sugars, 1 g protein.

SERVES 8

12 oz (350 g) silken tofu

¼ cup (60 mL) extra virgin olive oil

2 Tbsp (30 mL) fresh lemon juice

1 Tbsp (15 mL) honey

¼ cup (60 mL) finely chopped fresh dill

2 Tbsp (30 mL) minced sweet onion

3 Tbsp (45 mL) minced dill pickles (about 1 small pickle)

1 tsp (5 mL) Dijon mustard

½ tsp (2 mL) sea salt

⅛ tsp (0.5 mL) freshly ground black pepper

Sliced fresh vegetables, for dipping

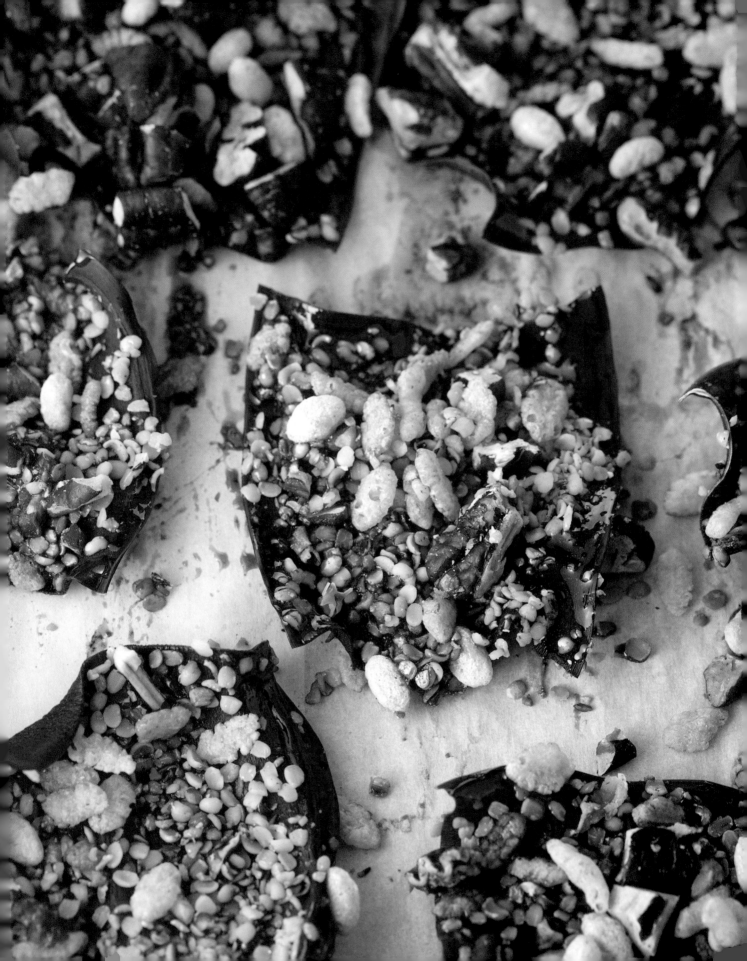

Salty-Sweet Kombu Chips

If you love kale chips, you have to try these kombu chips—a similar item made from a type of seaweed known as kombu instead of from leafy greens. Kombu, when baked, makes a nutritious version of a chip. The salty-savoury flavour from concentrated minerals combines well with the seeds, nuts and syrups in the recipe, and the kombu is the perfect chip base. —Nettie

1. Soak the kombu in cold water for 45 minutes. Drain. Cut each piece into a 2-inch (5 cm) square.

2. Preheat oven to 250°F (120°C).

3. In a small bowl, combine the rice syrup and maple syrup. Whisk until smooth. Baste the syrup mixture onto the kombu with a brush.

4. Place basted kombu on a baking sheet lined with parchment paper.

5. In a medium-sized bowl, combine hemp seeds, pecans and rice cereal. Sprinkle on top of kombu.

6. Bake for 1½ hours or until crisp. Allow to cool on rack for 5 minutes.

7. Store in airtight container for up to 5 days.

SERVES 10

2 oz (60 g) dried kombu pieces

⅓ cup (75 mL) rice syrup

⅓ cup (75 mL) maple syrup

¼ cup (60 mL) hemp seeds

½ cup (125 mL) pecans, chopped

½ cup (125 mL) crisp rice cereal

Tip: Sold in health food stores, kombu is about 2 inches (5 cm) wide, deep green or black and packaged in strips. They are preserved by drying and reconstituted through soaking, where they become smooth and leathery. But do not be misled; they are not tough in texture. Once soaked, kombu expands to about three times the size of its original dry state and resembles lasagne noodles.

NUTRIENTS PER SERVING SERVING SIZE: ¹⁄₁₀ RECIPE

146 calories, 8 g fat, 1 g saturated fat, 160 mg sodium, 17 g carbohydrates, 3 g fibre, 10 g sugars, 4 g protein. Good source of magnesium.

Curried Tomato & Lentil Dal Dip

Many people are familiar with curry powder, but not garam masala, which is a Northern Indian spice blend that includes some combination of cardamom, cloves, black peppercorns, cumin, cinnamon, nutmeg and mace. Unlike curry powder, which can be added at the beginning or end of a recipe, garam masala is meant to be used as a final seasoning at the end of a dish. Both curry powder and garam masala are wonderful additions to your spice pantry, and this recipe uses them in combination, offering a beautiful flavour profile. Serve this dip with whole grain pita triangles. —Nettie

1. In a medium-sized pot over medium heat, heat oil. Add the garlic and onions and cook for 5 minutes or until softened. Stir in lentils, water, curry powder, tomato paste, sugar and salt. Cook for 20–25 minutes or until lentils are soft.
2. Add yogurt. Stir well.
3. Remove from heat and stir in the garam masala. Sprinkle with cilantro. Serve warm immediately, or refrigerate and serve cool.

SERVES 10

2 Tbsp (30 mL) extra virgin olive oil

2 garlic cloves, minced

1 sweet onion, finely diced

1 cup (250 mL) dried red lentils

2 cups (500 mL) water

2 tsp (10 mL) curry powder

5½ oz (160 g) tomato paste

1 tsp (5 mL) brown sugar

½ tsp (2 mL) sea salt

½ cup (125 mL) 2% Greek yogurt

½ tsp (2 mL) garam masala

NUTRIENTS PER SERVING
SERVING SIZE: ¼ CUP (60 ML) DIP

106 calories, 3 g fat, 0.5 g saturated fat, 120 mg sodium, 15 g carbohydrates, 4 g fibre, 4 g sugars, 6 g protein. Good source of fibre and iron.

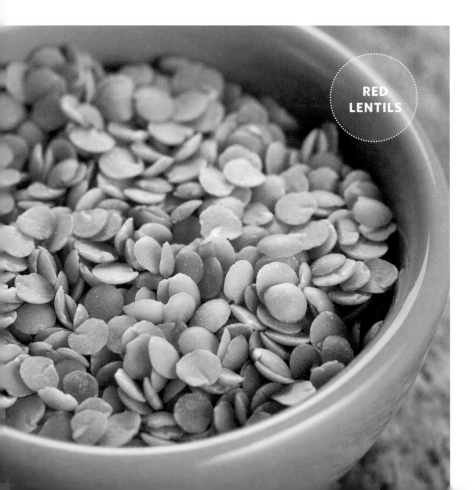

RED
LENTILS

Cashew Butter, Quinoa & Eggplant Dip

This lovely dip has a flavour profile similar to baba ghanouj, but has added texture from the quinoa. It's a perfect dip for your favourite crunchy vegetables, such as carrots, celery and peppers. —Nettie

1. Preheat the oven to broil and move the oven rack to top position.
2. In a medium pot over medium heat, add olive oil and sauté the onion and garlic for 5 minutes or until soft. Stir in the quinoa and lightly cook for 1 minute. Stir in broth and bring to a boil. Reduce heat, cover the pot and gently simmer for 15 minutes. Remove from heat and let stand for 5 minutes. Uncover, fluff with a fork and transfer to a medium bowl.
3. Pierce eggplant several times all over with a fork and place on baking sheet lined with parchment paper. Broil, turning occasionally, for 20 minutes or until the skins are browned and the centres soft. Skin will char and blister, and the flesh will collapse.
4. Transfer the eggplant to a cutting board. Let cool. Slice the eggplants in half lengthwise and scrape out the pulp.
5. In a food processor, purée eggplant pulp with parsley, cashew butter, soy sauce, lemon juice, salt and pepper.
6. Add eggplant mixture to the quinoa. Stir to combine. Serve, garnished with parsley.

SERVES 8

1 Tbsp (15 mL) extra virgin olive oil

1 onion, minced

2 garlic cloves, minced

1 cup (250 mL) quinoa, rinsed

2 cups (500 mL) no-salt-added vegetable broth

1 medium eggplant

½ cup (125 mL) chopped fresh parsley

½ cup (125 mL) cashew butter

1½ Tbsp (22 mL) sodium-reduced soy sauce

2 Tbsp (30 mL) fresh lemon juice

¼ tsp (1 mL) sea salt

⅛ tsp (0.5 mL) freshly ground black pepper

NUTRIENTS PER SERVING
SERVING SIZE: ¼ CUP (60 ML) DIP

109 calories, 6 g fat, 1 g saturated fat, 91 mg sodium, 13 g carbohydrates, 2 g fibre, 2 g sugars, 4 g protein. Good source of folate and magnesium.

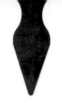

Spice-Roasted Chickpeas

Roasted chickpeas are so addictive and are a perfect snack or appetizer when combined with nuts and seeds. The reason we specifically recommend kosher salt in this recipe is because its coarse texture will add more of a crunch than the fine granules found in fine sea salt. This is a snack food, after all—you want to taste some salt! —Cara

1. Preheat the oven to 400°F
2. In a medium bowl, combine the chickpeas, oil, cumin, paprika, salt and pepper. Spread out in a single layer on a baking sheet lined wirh parchment paper and roast for about 30 minutes, stirring once or twice.
3. Add the almonds, stir and roast for another 10 minutes. Add sunflower and pumpkin seeds. Roast for 5–10 more minutes until brown and crisp. Remove from oven and pour into a medium-sized bowl. Season with extra salt, if needed, and serve immediately.

A Note About Salt

If you are watching your salt intake, switching the type of salt you use is not the answer. Table salt, sea salt and kosher salt are all the same chemical compound—sodium chloride. They differ in shape, size and structure, but are all essentially salt. And all have virtually the same amount of sodium. If you want to cut back on sodium, the best way to do that is to cut back on your intake of processed foods and fast food, which is where most of the salt in the diet comes from. (See salt sidebar, page 126.)

SERVES 6

14 oz (410 mL) can no-salt-added chickpeas, rinsed and drained

¼ cup (60 mL) extra virgin olive oil

1 tsp (5 mL) ground cumin

1 tsp (5 mL) paprika

1 tsp (5 mL) kosher salt

½ tsp (2 mL) freshly ground black pepper

1 cup (250 mL) raw unsalted almonds, halved

¼ cup (60 mL) raw unsalted sunflower seeds

¼ cup (60 mL) raw unsalted pumpkin seeds

NUTRIENTS PER SERVING SERVING SIZE: ¼ CUP (60 ML)

261 calories, 20 g fat, 2 g saturated fat, 208 mg sodium, 14 g carbohydrates, 5 g fibre, 1 g sugars, 8 g protein. High in fibre. Excellent source of vitamin E, magnesium and manganese. Good source of folate, zinc and copper.

Tempeh Pâté

If you love chopped liver and foie gras, the flavour profile of this pâté will please your palate. I have been using tempeh to replace chicken and beef for over 30 years, and I love its taste and texture. It has a firm, chewy texture and adds a meaty layer to recipes. The fermentation process enhances the flavour and makes the protein in the soybean easier to digest. Enjoy this pâté on the Sunflower Barley Crackers (page 75). —Nettie

SERVES 8

1 cup (250 mL) raw unsalted almonds

2 Tbsp (30 mL) extra virgin olive oil

1 onion, diced

2 garlic cloves, minced

2 cups (500 mL) sliced button mushrooms

½ lb (225 g) tempeh, fresh or thawed, cut into ½-inch (1 cm) cubes

1 tsp (5 mL) sodium-reduced tamari

½ tsp (2 mL) dried thyme

½ tsp (2 mL) dried sage

½ cup (125 mL) chopped fresh dill

¼ tsp (1 mL) sea salt

1. Preheat oven to 350°F (180°C). Spread almonds on a baking sheet lined with parchment paper and bake until golden, about 5 minutes.

2. In a medium-sized saucepan, heat olive oil over medium heat. Add onion and garlic, and sauté 5 minutes or until soft. Add mushrooms and sauté for 3–5 minutes.

3. Add tempeh to the vegetable mixture. Stir to combine. Add tamari, thyme, sage, dill and salt. Cook 12–15 minutes or until most of liquid has evaporated.

4. In a food processor, grind almonds. Add cooked mushroom mixture and process until pâté is thick and smooth. Cover and chill for at least 30 minutes.

5. Serve with cut vegetables and whole grain crackers.

Tip: Find tempeh in the fridge or freezer at the grocery store or health food store. Always check expiry date on fresh tempeh and keep it refrigerated. Tempeh can be frozen for a maximum of 6 months.

NUTRIENTS PER SERVING
SERVING SIZE: 2 TBSP (30 ML) PÂTÉ

162 calories, 12 g fat, 2 g saturated fat, 106 mg sodium, 7 g carbohydrates, 2 g fibre, 2 g sugars, 8 g protein. Good source of riboflavin and magnesium.

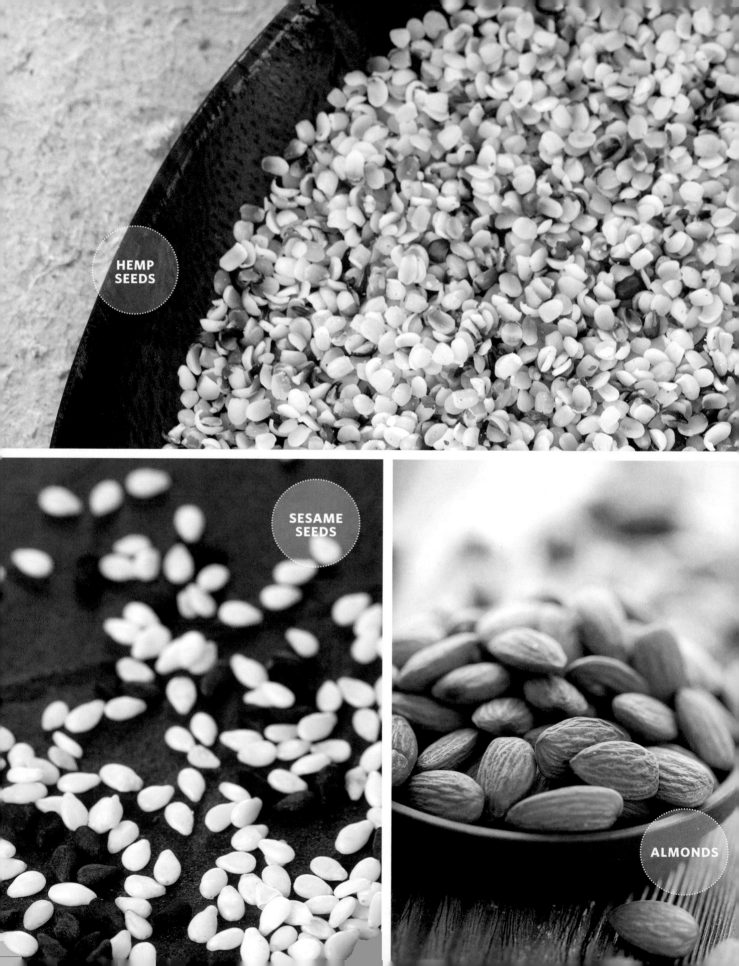

HEMP
SEEDS

SESAME
SEEDS

ALMONDS

Crunchy Seed & Nut Butter

Pastes made from finely ground nuts or seeds are referred to as "butters." Tahini is a thick, smooth paste made of hulled and ground sesame seeds. I especially like to combine peanut butter and tahini together because they have a rich, satisfying taste. The nuts and seeds add extra crunch, reminiscent of chunky peanut butter. Serve on toast or crackers, spread on pancakes, swirl into yogurt or use it wherever you'd use peanut butter! —Nettie

1. Preheat the oven to 350°F (180°C).
2. Spread out hemp seeds, sesame seeds and almonds on a baking sheet lined with parchment paper. Toast in oven for 3–5 minutes, turning once, until golden brown. Allow to cool.
3. In a small bowl, mix together the toasted seeds and almonds, peanut butter, tahini and honey until well combined.
4. Serve with crackers, as a sandwich spread, on oatmeal or as a vegetable dip.

 Tip: If you prefer a smooth texture in your nut butter, grind the toasted hemp seeds, sesame seeds and almonds in a spice grinder before adding them to the peanut butter and tahini.

 Tip: For a chai-inspired seed and nut butter, prepare this recipe with the Chai-Spiced Honey on page 35.

SERVES 8

3 Tbsp (45 mL) hemp seeds

3 Tbsp (45 mL) sesame seeds

3 Tbsp (45 mL) chopped unsalted almonds

½ cup (125 mL) smooth natural peanut butter

¼ cup (60 mL) tahini

½ tsp (2 mL) honey

NUTRIENTS PER SERVING
SERVING SIZE: 2 TBSP (30 ML) NUT BUTTER

164 calories, 14 g fat, 2 g saturated fat, 22 mg sodium, 6 g carbohydrates, 2 g fibre, 2 g sugars, 6 g protein.

Spicy-Sweet Toasted Seeds

This is the perfect recipe to prepare for last-minute guests, when time is tight but you want to make something impressive. You may want to double this recipe when company is coming; it's always well-enjoyed. In a pinch, the same spice blend will work equally well on almonds, walnuts or pecans too. —Cara

1. In a heavy skillet, heat the olive oil over medium heat. Add the pumpkin and sunflower seeds and stir frequently, until they are evenly toasted and begin to pop, about 5 minutes.

2. Stir in the sugar, salt, cumin, chili powder and cinnamon and cook, stirring constantly, for 1–2 minutes, or until well-blended.

3. Transfer to a serving bowl and serve with a spoon, so guests can serve themselves small handfuls.

NUTRIENTS PER SERVING
SERVING SIZE: ¼ CUP (60 ML) SEEDS

222 calories, 20 g fat, 3 g saturated fat, 295 mg sodium, 7 g carbohydrates, 3 g fibre, 2 g sugars, 9 g protein. Excellent source of thiamin, vitamin E, magnesium, zinc, manganese and copper. Good source of vitamin B$_6$, folate and iron.

SERVES 8

1 Tbsp (15 mL) extra virgin olive oil

1 cup (250 mL) raw unsalted pumpkin seeds

1 cup (250 mL) raw unsalted sunflower seeds

2 tsp (10 mL) granulated sugar

1 tsp (5 mL) kosher salt

½ tsp (2 mL) ground cumin

½ tsp (2 mL) chili powder

¼ tsp (1 mL) ground cinnamon

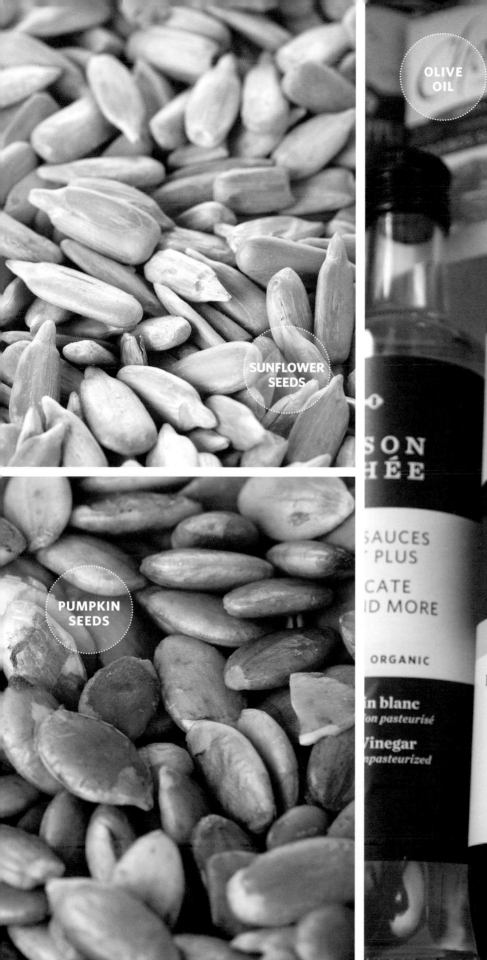

SUNFLOWER SEEDS

PUMPKIN SEEDS

OLIVE OIL

MAISON ORPHÉE

POUR LA CUISINE AU QUOTIDIEN

FOR EVERYDAY COOKING

BIOLOGIQUE ❦ ORGANIC

Huile d'olive extra vierge
Extraction à froid

Extra-Virgin Olive Oil
Cold Extraction

DÉLICATE • DELICATE

(16.9 fl oz) 500 ml

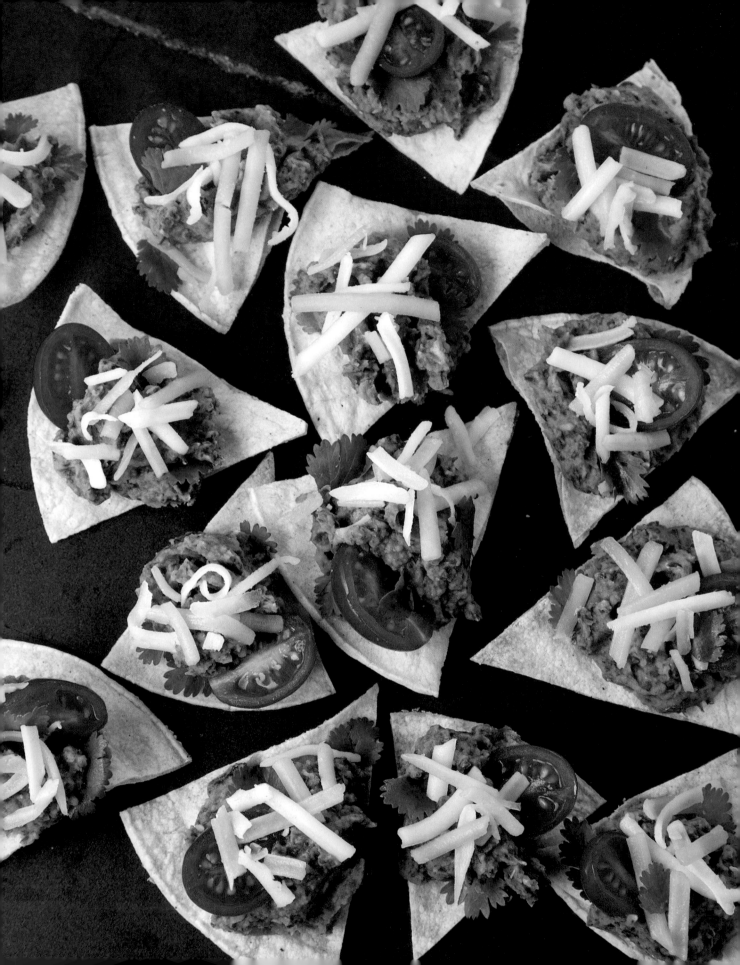

Picante Black Bean Dip on Corn Tortilla Chips

I love having a combination of bold flavours in one bite-sized taste. This appetizer has the right blend of crunchy, salty, tart and spicy. You can serve individually dressed tortilla chips as indicated below, or serve it nacho-style for a large group. —Cara

1. Preheat oven to 350°F (180°C). Place corn tortilla triangles on baking sheet lined with parchment paper. Bake until edges brown, about 10 minutes. Remove and allow to cool. (They will get crunchy as they cool.)

2. In a food processor, add beans, onion, cilantro, garlic, oregano, cumin, paprika, cayenne, lime juice and salt. Purée until smooth.

3. Add 1 tsp (5 mL) of black bean spread to each tortilla. Top with cheese.

4. Serve, garnished with cilantro and grape tomatoes.

 Tip: If you can't find corn tortillas, use whole wheat tortillas instead.

NUTRIENTS PER SERVING SERVING SIZE: 6 TRIANGLES

155 calories, 3 g fat, 1½ g saturated fat, 48 mg sodium, 24 g carbohydrates, 4½ g fibre, 1½ g sugars, 6 g protein.

SERVES 8

8 soft corn tortillas (4 inch/10 cm), each cut into 6 triangles

19 oz can (560 mL) no-salt-added black beans, drained and rinsed

1 red onion, minced

3 Tbsp (45 mL) minced fresh cilantro

1 garlic clove, minced

½ tsp (2 mL) dried oregano

1 tsp (5 mL) ground cumin

½ tsp (2 mL) smoked paprika

⅛ tsp (0.5 mL) cayenne pepper

2 tsp (10 mL) fresh lime juice

¼ tsp (1 mL) sea salt

½ cup (125 mL) shredded cheddar cheese

¼ cup (60 mL) chopped fresh cilantro leaves, for garnish

½ cup (125 mL) grape tomato halves, for garnish

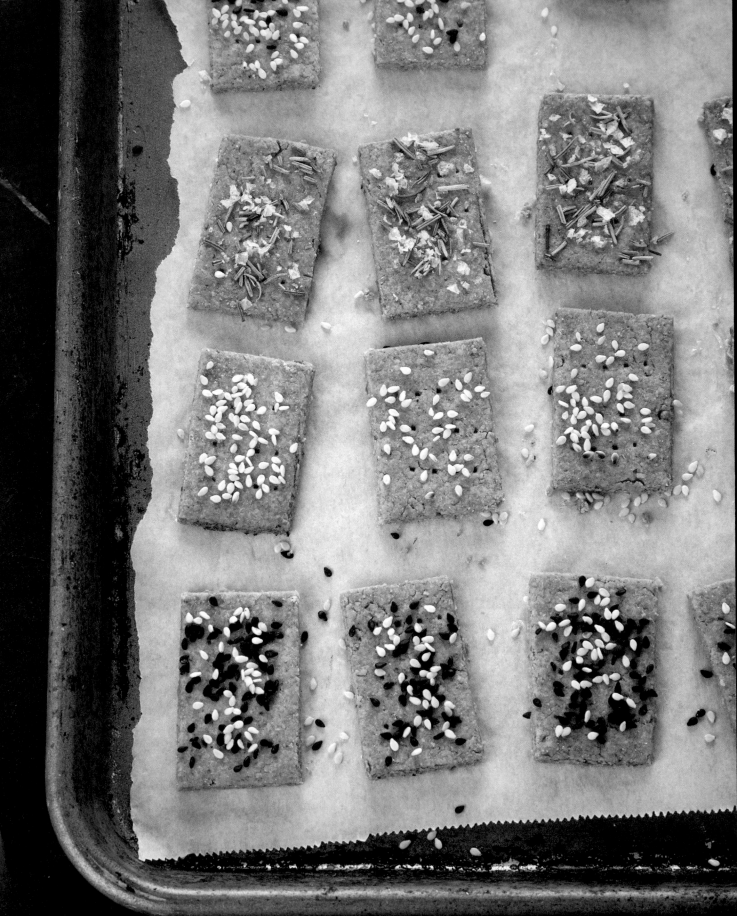

Sunflower Barley Crackers

These simple crackers are perfect for topping with spreads, dips or cheeses. It's not easy to find packaged crackers where the first ingredient is anything other than enriched wheat flour, so these are a nice departure from store-bought crackers and easy to make. Most grocery stores now carry barley flour—we like the ones made by Bob's Red Mill or Oak Manor. We purposely left the flavour profile plain, so these crackers can be dressed up by using your imagination. For a suggestion on how to jazz them up, see the tip below. —Cara

1. Preheat oven to 350°F (180°F).

2. In a medium bowl, combine barley flour, salt, sunflower seeds, hemp seeds and oil. Gradually add just enough water to form a soft dough. Knead dough and roll out on a lightly floured surface to ⅛-inch (3 mm) thickness.

3. Cut into rectangles and prick each cracker several times with a folk. Arrange on a baking sheet lined with parchment paper. Bake for 10 minutes or until lightly browned.

4. Serve with your favourite dips or cheeses.

Tip: If you are planning to use the crackers for dipping, keep them plain. That way, the dip will be the prominent flavour. If the crackers are the star, you can sprinkle them before baking with toppings like sesame seeds, poppy seeds, dried rosemary and sea salt, cracked black pepper, or smoked paprika. Just brush the unbaked crackers with lightly beaten egg white before adding the toppings to help them stick.

MAKES 24 CRACKERS

1 cup (250 mL) whole barley flour

¼ tsp (1 mL) sea salt

¼ cup (60 mL) raw unsalted sunflower seeds, finely ground

¼ cup (60 mL) hemp seeds, finely ground

3 Tbsp (45 mL) extra virgin olive oil

3 Tbsp (45 mL) water

NUTRIENTS PER SERVING
SERVING SIZE: 2 CRACKERS

126 calories, 7 g fat, 1 g saturated fat, 59 mg sodium, 12 g carbohydrates, 2 g fibre, 0 g sugars, 4 g protein.

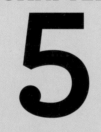

CHAPTER

5

Salads

Tip: Edamame is a Japanese term for young soybeans (literal translation: stem beans), the still-green baby beans inside the pod. They are a super source of protein—1 cup (250 mL) contains a whopping 23 grams, rivalling a 2.5 ounce chicken breast, salmon fillet or sirloin steak.

Edamame Salad with Carrot-Ginger Dressing

My friend Erik is a born-and-raised New Yorker, and whenever I'm in the city we make time to meet up. Back in 2005, we shared a memorable dinner at the Sidewalk Café in the East Village. His favourite item on the menu was their signature salad dressing—a zesty, bright-orange concoction with a tangy bite. He enjoyed its complexity and balance of flavours, which I detected to be ginger, carrot and soy sauce. I promised I'd develop a recipe for him based on that wonderful dressing, and this, finally, is it. I hope it's worth the wait.   Cara

1. In a small pot, bring water to a boil. Add edamame and cook about 5 minutes. Drain and allow to cool.

2. In a large bowl, add greens, avocado, cucumber, tomatoes and edamame.

3. To prepare the dressing, combine oil, vinegar, tamari, ginger, carrots, onion, sugar and salt in a food processor or blender, and process until smooth.

4. Add ¾ cup (175 mL) of the dressing to the bowl of greens and vegetables, and toss until evenly coated; serve immediately.

> **Tip:** This recipe makes about 1½ cups of dressing; you will likely only use ¾ cup (175 mL) on the salad. Unused dressing will keep for up to two weeks in the refrigerator.

NUTRIENTS PER SERVING SERVING SIZE: ⅙ RECIPE

193 calories, 15 g fat, 2 g saturated fat, 249 mg sodium, 11 g carbohydrates, 5 g fibre, 4 g sugars, 5 g protein. High in fibre. Excellent source of vitamin A and folate. Good source of vitamin C and magnesium.

SERVES 6

1 cup (250 mL) frozen shelled edamame beans

6 cups (1.5 L) mixed greens

1 ripe avocado, diced

½ English cucumber, diced

1 cup (250 mL) cherry tomatoes, halved

Dressing

½ cup (125 mL) extra virgin olive oil

¼ cup (60 mL) rice vinegar

2 Tbsp (30 mL) sodium-reduced tamari

1 tsp (5 mL) finely grated ginger

1 carrot, diced

1 tsp (5 mL) diced Vidalia or other sweet onion

1½ tsp (2 mL) granulated sugar

Pinch of sea salt

Carrot & Kohlrabi Slaw

The bright flavours in this tasty slaw come from the wonderful spices, which include garam masala—a ready-made spice blend of cinnamon, cumin, coriander, pepper, cardamom and cloves. It's fragrant and flavourful but not spicy, and this salad is my daughter Kasey's favourite way to eat carrots! Part of the cabbage family, kohlrabi is a mild-flavoured root with bitter leafy green stalks—and both parts are edible. This recipe uses only the gentle and subtle flavour of the root, which is high in fibre and vitamin C. —Cara

1. In a large bowl, add carrots, kohlrabi, raisins, almonds and hemp seeds.
2. In a small bowl, whisk together the oil, vinegar, cumin, cinnamon and garam masala. Add salt and pepper. Stir to combine.
3. Pour dressing over slaw. Toss well and enjoy.

For tips on toasting nuts and seeds, see page 25.

Tip: Rice wine vinegar is mild vinegar that is naturally sweet. Avoid "seasoned" rice wine vinegar. It contains unnecessary added sugar.

NUTRIENTS PER SERVING

SERVING SIZE: 1½ CUPS (375 ML) SLAW

187 calories, 14 g fat, 1 g saturated fat, 80 mg sodium, 13 g carbohydrates, 4 g fibre, 7 g sugars, 4 g protein. High in fibre. Excellent source of vitamin A. Good source of vitamin C.

SERVES 6

6 carrots, grated

4 kohlrabi bulbs, peeled and grated

½ cup (125 mL) raisins

½ cup (125 mL) slivered almonds, toasted

¼ cup (60 mL) hemp seeds, toasted

Dressing

½ cup (125 mL) extra virgin olive oil

¼ cup (60 mL) unseasoned rice wine vinegar

2 tsp (10 mL) ground cumin

1 tsp (5 mL) ground cinnamon

1 tsp (5 mL) garam masala

¼ tsp (1 mL) sea salt

¼ tsp (1 mL) freshly ground black pepper

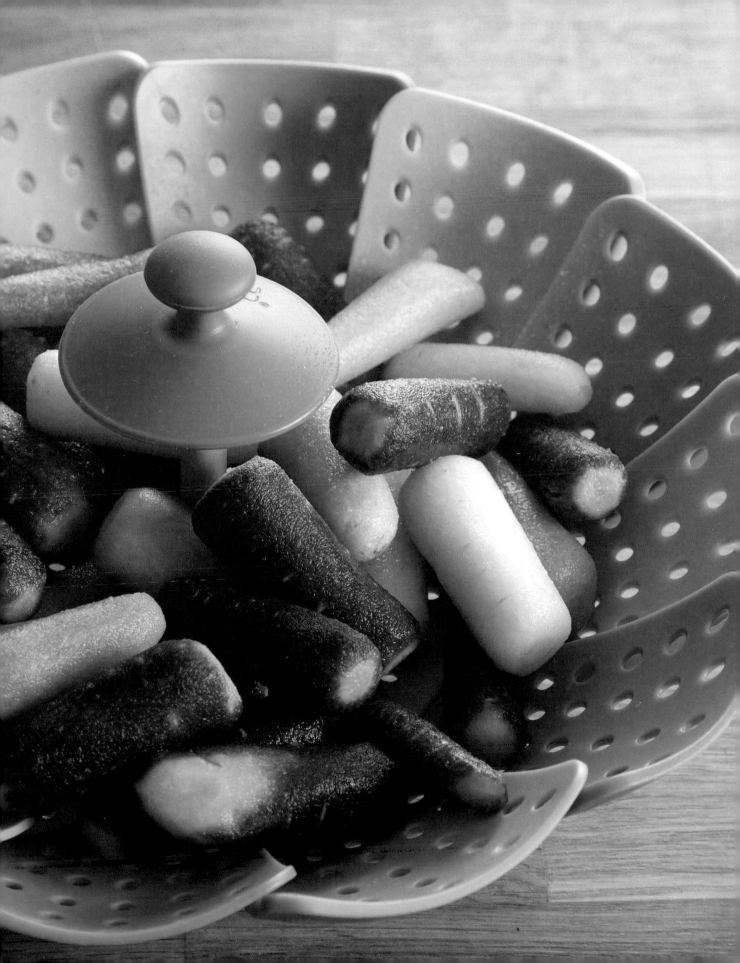

Almond Fennel Celery Slaw

Do you eat with your eyes first? Or is texture your number one requirement when enjoying a meal? I am happy to report that this recipe has wonderful colour, texture and flavour! The crisp taste from the apple combined with the crunch of celery and fennel allows the sweet, mild taste of the orange to fill your mouth with a symphony of flavour. Purple, orange, green and white, this salad is visually appealing too. —Nettie

1. Place the fennel, cabbage, celery, apple, orange, beans and basil in a large salad bowl. Toss well.
2. In a medium-sized bowl, whisk together vinegar, mustard, honey, salt and pepper. Slowly whisk in the oil until well combined.
3. Add dressing to the slaw mixture and toss well. Add almonds to garnish.

 Tip: You can also use green cabbage in this recipe, but the red variety has a slight edge in terms of superfood potential. It's high in anthocyanin, an antioxidant found in red, blue and purple vegetables that's known for its potential anti-inflammatory effect.

NUTRIENTS PER SERVING
SERVING SIZE: 1½ CUPS (375 ML) SLAW

187 calories, 14 g fat, 1 g saturated fat, 80 mg sodium, 13 g carbohydrates, 4 g fibre, 7 g sugars, 4 g protein. High in fibre. Excellent source of vitamin A. Good source of vitamin C.

SERVES 6

1 fennel bulb, thinly sliced

½ medium red cabbage, thinly sliced

3 celery stalks, thinly sliced

1 large Fuji apple, thinly sliced

1 medium orange, peeled and sliced into 1-inch (2.5 cm) pieces

14 oz (410 mL) can of no-salt-added cannellini beans, drained and rinsed

¼ cup (60 mL) chopped fresh basil

Dressing

¼ cup (60 mL) apple cider vinegar

2 tsp (10 mL) Dijon mustard

1 tsp (5 mL) honey

¼ tsp (1 mL) sea salt

⅛ tsp (0.5 mL) freshly ground pepper

¼ cup (60 mL) extra virgin olive oil

½ cup (125 mL) almonds, chopped and toasted (see page 25), for garnish

Celery Salad with Lemon Dressing

You're probably familiar with celery stalks, but the leaves are edible too, and are so delicious! Celery has a close cousin called celery root or celeriac—it has the same flavour profile. Layering these three ingredients deepens the flavour of this bright, fresh salad. And, it's even better the next day—it retains the phenomenal crunch while absorbing more of the lemony flavour. —Cara

SERVES 6

6 stalks celery, thinly sliced

3 celery leaves, thinly sliced (choose sweet inner leaves)

1 medium bulb celery root, peeled and thinly sliced

2 small golden or candy cane beets, peeled and thinly sliced

¼ cup (60 mL) dried apricots

¼ cup (60 mL) unsalted sunflower seeds, toasted (see page 25)

Zest of 1 small lemon

Dressing

¼ cup (60 mL) extra virgin olive oil

2 Tbsp (30 mL) fresh lemon juice

1 tsp (5 mL) Dijon mustard

½ tsp (2 mL) honey

¼ tsp (1 mL) sea salt

⅛ tsp (0.5 mL) freshly ground black pepper

1. In a large bowl, combine celery stalks, leaves and roots; beets; apricots; seeds; and lemon zest. Stir to combine.

2. In a small bowl, whisk together olive oil, lemon juice, mustard and honey. Add salt and pepper.

3. Add dressing to celery salad and toss well.

Tip: If you have a mandolin, use it to thinly slice the celery stalks, celery root and beets. Mandolins are very handy kitchen tools to have—they transforms vegetables into perfectly uniform slices in seconds. While master-quality mandolins can cost upwards of a $100, you can also use a simple hand-held version, which you can buy, for about $15. Be careful with them, though; they are very sharp.

NUTRIENTS PER SERVING
SERVING SIZE: 1 CUP (250 ML) SALAD

169 calories, 12 g fat, 2 g saturated fat, 211 mg sodium, 15 g carbohydrates, 3 g fibre, 10 g sugars, 2 g protein. Good source of folate.

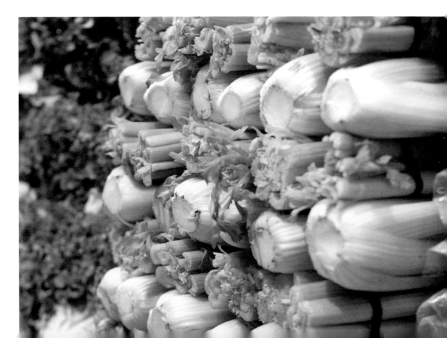

Tofu Caprese Stack

Fresh and bursting with flavour, these stacks are a good introduction to extra firm tofu, a neutral-tasting soy food. Tofu absorbs the flavours of the vinaigrette beautifully. The presentation of this dish is lovely; it makes a great appetizer salad when company is coming. —Nettie

1. To make the vinaigrette, in a small bowl, whisk together lime juice, vinegar, mustard and shallot.

2. Slowly add the olive oil in a thin stream, whisking constantly.

3. Add salt and pepper. Whisk to combine. Set vinaigrette aside.

4. To make the salad, cut each tomato into six horizontal slices.

5. Cut each tofu block vertically into ¼-inch (6 mm) slices (you should have 8 slices from 2 blocks of tofu).

6. Using a 3-inch (7.5 cm) round cookie cutter, cut 8 rounds from the tofu slices, reserving scraps for another use.

7. To serve, using four salad plates, place one slice of tomato in the centre of each plate. Top each slice of tomato with tofu and a basil leaf. Drizzle one-third of vinaigrette over the tofu, divided evenly among the plates. Top with a piece of bocconcini.

8. Repeat step 7 two more times to use up remaining tomatoes, tofu, basil, vinaigrette and bocconcini.

9. Marinate salad for 30 minutes (optional).

 Tip: Once opened, tofu will last for five days in your refrigerator. To store unused tofu, put it in a container and cover it with cold water and a lid. Change the water daily. Leftover tofu can also be frozen, or used in chili, stir-fries, pasta sauce or in salads.

SERVES 4

Vinaigrette

Juice of ½ lime (about 1 Tbsp/15 mL)

1 tsp (5 mL) balsamic vinegar

2 tsp (10 mL) Dijon mustard

1 small shallot, minced

3 Tbsp (45 mL) extra virgin olive oil

¼ tsp (1 mL) sea salt

⅛ tsp (0.5 mL) freshly ground black pepper

Salad

2 large tomatoes

2 packages (12 oz/350 g each) extra firm tofu, drained and rinsed

12 large fresh basil leaves

6 large-sized (2 inch/5 cm) bocconcini cheese rounds, sliced in half

NUTRIENTS PER SERVING SERVING SIZE: 1 STACK

390 calories, 29 g fat, 8 g saturated fat, 233 mg sodium, 7 g carbohydrates, 1 g fibre, 2 g sugars, 27 g protein. Excellent source of calcium and iron.

Black Bean & Quinoa Salad with Charred Corn

The best way to char corn is on the barbeque, but the cold-weather solution is to use a cast iron skillet. That's what we did for this recipe, and the results were perfect. Charring brings out a smoky sweetness in the corn and adds a wonderful layer of flavour to this robust salad. The unity between corn, cilantro, lime and cumin is a thing of beauty. —Cara

1. In a medium-sized saucepan, combine quinoa and broth. Bring to a boil, then simmer, covered, for 15 minutes. Let stand for 5 minutes, then fluff with a fork. Transfer to a large serving bowl.

2. In a heavy skillet on your stovetop, toast corn kernels over high heat until charred, about 8 minutes. Set aside to cool.

3. Add black beans, corn, yellow pepper, tomato, mango, onion and cilantro to quinoa. Stir to combine.

4. To make the dressing, in a small bowl, combine oil, lime juice, cumin, honey, garlic and salt. Whisk to combine.

5. Pour dressing over quinoa and toss to coat. Serve and enjoy.

Tip: You can use fresh, frozen or canned corn niblets in this recipe, but the frozen are the easiest and most convenient. They can go straight from the freezer right into the hot skillet.

SERVES 6

½ cup (125 mL) quinoa, rinsed

1 cup (250 mL) no-salt-added vegetable broth

1 cup (250 mL) frozen corn kernels

14 oz (410 mL) can no-salt-added black beans, drained

1 yellow pepper, seeded and diced

1 medium tomato, diced

1 mango, diced into ½-inch (1 cm) cubes

¼ red onion, finely diced

½ cup (125 mL) chopped fresh cilantro

Dressing

⅓ cup (75 mL) extra virgin olive oil

¼ cup (60 mL) fresh lime juice

1 tsp (5 mL) ground cumin

1 tsp (5 mL) honey

1 garlic clove, crushed

½ tsp (2 mL) sea salt

NUTRIENTS PER SERVING
SERVING SIZE: 1 CUP (250 ML) SALAD

340 calories, 19 g fat, 3 g saturated fat, 17 mg sodium, 37 g carbohydrates, 6 g fibre, 9 g sugars, 8 g protein. Very high in fibre. Excellent source of folate, vitamin C and magnesium. Good source of iron.

Warm French Lentil & Potato Salad

This salad can be prepared two ways: with or without bacon. Guess which I prefer? —Nettie

1. If using, in a large skillet, cook bacon over medium-high heat, turning once until browned and crisp or for 7–10 minutes. Use a slotted spoon or tongs, transfer bacon to a paper towel–lined plate and let drain. Coarsely chop and set aside.

2. In a large saucepan, add lentils, onion, thyme, carrot and bay leaf. Add stock and bring to a boil. Lower heat to simmer. Cook until lentils are tender, 25–30 minutes. Drain and discard bay leaf.

3. Bring a large pot of water to a boil over high heat. Add the potatoes in their skins, cover and reduce the heat to medium-low. Cook until tender, about 12 minutes.

4. To make dressing, in a small bowl, add shallot and vinegar; let stand for 5 minutes. Add garlic, salt, pepper and mustard. Whisk in the olive oil to make a thick dressing.

5. To serve, dress the lentils with one-third of the dressing, then transfer to a platter or serving bowl. Arrange potatoes cut side up around the lentils. Add bacon on top of lentils, if using. Add the chopped capers and cornichons on top. Pour the remaining vinaigrette over. Sprinkle with parsley and chives.

 Tip: Bacon adds tons of flavour, but also increases the fat, calorie and sodium content.

NUTRIENTS PER SERVING
SERVING SIZE: 1 CUP (250 ML) SALAD

With bacon: 368 calories, 15 g fat, 3 g saturated fat, 521 mg sodium, 48 g carbohydrates, 10 g fibre, 7 g sugars, 13 g protein. Very high in fibre. Excellent source of vitamin C, vitamin K and iron. Good source of vitamin A.

Without bacon: 314 calories, 10 g fat, 1 g saturated fat, 290 mg sodium, 48 g carbohydrates, 10 g fibre, 7 g sugars, 13 g protein. Excellent source of vitamin B$_{12}$. Good source of riboflavin, folate, calcium and zinc.

SERVES 6

½ lb (225 g) bacon (optional)

1½ cups (500 mL) green lentils, rinsed

1 onion, thinly sliced

½ tsp (2 mL) dried thyme

1 carrot, grated

1 small bay leaf

4 cups (1 L) no-salt-added vegetable stock

1 lb (450 g) fingerling or other small potatoes, rinsed and halved

Dressing

1 large shallot, finely diced

2 Tbsp (30 mL) red wine vinegar

2 garlic cloves, minced

⅛ tsp (0.5 mL) sea salt

⅛ tsp (0.5 mL) freshly ground black pepper

1 Tbsp (15 mL) Dijon mustard

¼ cup (60 mL) extra virgin olive oil

Toppings

2 tsp (10 mL) capers, rinsed and chopped

2 Tbsp (30 mL) chopped cornichons or sour pickle

½ cup (125 mL) chopped fresh parsley

¼ cup (60 mL) chopped fresh chives

Tip: The vitamin C in the strawberries helps your body absorb the iron from the kale. Another great fruit and vegetable pairing is spinach with mandarin oranges.

Strawberry Kale Salad with Garam Masala–Spiced Seeds

Pairing kale with strawberries and maple syrup cuts the bitter edge off this leafy green, leaving every bite with the perfect sweet-savoury flavour profile. If I want to entice my kids into eating kale, this is the go-to salad that I make. Sometimes we crumble goat cheese on top. According to my daughter Kasey, everything is better with cheese! —Cara

1. In a small saucepan over medium heat, toast pumpkin seeds with maple syrup and garam masala for about 7 minutes, or until coated and fragrant. Set aside to cool on a plate.

2. In a large bowl, add kale and strawberries. Add the pumpkin seeds once they have cooled to room temperature.

3. To make dressing, whisk together oil, vinegar, syrup, mustard and mint.

4. Add ½ cup (125 mL) of dressing to lightly coat salad and toss well. Serve immediately.

Note: There will be some leftover dressing. Store in a jar with a tight-fitting lid and refrigerate for up to 1 week.

 Tip: Baby kale is a small-sized leafy green that you can purchase in the salad section—it comes in a bag or plastic container. It's similar to baby spinach or mixed spring greens, which can also be used in this recipe if you can't find baby kale.

SERVES 6

½ cup (125 mL) raw unsalted pumpkin seeds

2 tsp (10 mL) pure maple syrup

1 tsp (5 mL) garam masala

6 cups (1.5 L) baby kale

2 cups (500 mL) sliced and hulled strawberries

Dressing

½ cup (125 mL) extra virgin olive oil

¼ cup (60 mL) balsamic vinegar

1 tsp (5 mL) pure maple syrup

1 Tbsp (15 mL) Dijon mustard

1 Tbsp (15 mL) chopped fresh mint

NUTRIENTS PER SERVING
SERVING SIZE: 1⅓ CUPS (320 ML) SALAD

226 calories, 16 g fat, 2 g saturated fat, 105 mg sodium, 18 g carbohydrates, 5 g fibre, 5 g sugars, 7 g protein. Excellent source of vitamin A and vitamin C. Good source of folate, calcium and iron.

Leek & Lentil Salad

Quick-cooking lentils are the only legume that do not need to be soaked before they are boiled, making them a quick and easy ingredient to work with. Flavourful and hearty, I enjoy this recipe hot or cold, and often stuff this salad into a whole wheat pita for an easy, portable meal on the go. —Nettie

1. Heat 2 Tbsp (30 mL) oil in a large pot over medium heat. Sauté leeks and garlic for 3–5 minutes or until softened. Sprinkle with ¼ tsp (1 mL) salt and ⅛ tsp (1 mL) pepper.

2. Add the leek mixture to a large bowl, and toss with cilantro and vinegar. Set aside.

3. Heat the remaining 1 Tbsp (15 mL) oil in the large pot over high heat. Add onions and cook, stirring frequently for 5 minutes or until softened. Add peppers and cook, stirring until soft, for 3–5 minutes, and then add broth, lentils, cumin and paprika. Reduce heat to medium-low and simmer until the lentils are tender, about 30 minutes.

4. Stir in the remaining ¼ tsp (1 mL) salt and ⅛ tsp (1 mL) pepper. Spoon lentils into serving bowls and top with leek mixture before serving.

SERVES 6

3 Tbsp (45 mL) extra virgin olive oil, divided

2 leeks, thinly sliced (white and pale green parts only)

2 garlic cloves, minced

½ tsp (2 mL) sea salt, divided

¼ tsp (1 mL) freshly ground black pepper, divided

½ cup (125 mL) chopped fresh cilantro leaves

1 Tbsp (15 mL) apple cider vinegar

1 onion, finely diced

1 red pepper, finely diced

4 cups (1 L) no-salt-added vegetable broth

2 cups (500 mL) dried green, brown or black lentils, rinsed

1 tsp (5 mL) ground cumin

1 tsp (5 mL) smoked paprika

Tip: Red lentils (which are orange in colour—go figure!) cook in about 20–25 minutes and lose their disc shape; they become creamy and porridge-like. Green, brown and black lentils, which you can use interchangeably in this recipe, take about 25–35 minutes to cook and hold their disc shape nicely. Red lentils won't work in this recipe—if you use them, it'll be a messy porridge salad!

NUTRIENTS PER SERVING SERVING SIZE: 1 CUP (250 ML) SALAD

179 calories, 7 g fat, 1 g saturated fat, 304 mg sodium, 23 g carbohydrates, 5 g fibre, 7 g sugars, 5 g protein. High in fibre. Excellent source of vitamin C. Good source of vitamin A, folate and iron.

Roasted Tomato & Bean Salad

The roasting of tomatoes brings out a mellow sweetness, which makes this salad melt in your mouth. You can use green, yellow or purple beans in this recipe. Look for beans that are crisp, with no brown spots. If you store them in a plastic bag in the refrigerator, make sure to poke some holes in the plastic bag so they will stay fresh for longer. Purple beans turn green when cooked. Imagine my surprise the first time that happened! Don't be surprised when it happens to you too. —Nettie

1. Preheat oven to 375°F (190°C).
2. Place tomatoes on rimmed baking sheet lined with parchment paper and sprinkle the tomatoes with salt. Bake for at least 30 minutes until the tops begin to slightly brown. Set aside.
3. Add an inch (2.5 cm) of water to a pot, and place a steamer basket on top. Add beans and a tight-fitting lid, and steam about 5 minutes or until beans are tender crisp. Drain, pat dry and cut into ¼-inch (6 mm) pieces.
4. In a medium-sized skillet, heat oil over medium heat. Add shallots and sauté for 3–5 minutes until translucent. Add mushrooms and corn. Sauté for an additional 3 minutes until mushrooms are soft. Remove from heat. Transfer contents to a large bowl and add aduki beans and dill. Toss well.
5. Add roasted tomatoes and green beans. Stir to combine.
6. To make dressing, in a small bowl, combine the oil, lime juice, vinegar, mustard, salt and pepper. Whisk together. Pour onto salad and toss until evenly coated.
7. Divide salad greens among 6 plates. Add roasted tomato salad on top of greens.

 Tip: To retain more nutrients in the green beans, it's better to steam instead of boil them. Steaming cooks vegetables without submersing them in water, so they are more likely to retain vitamins and minerals.

SERVES 6

Salad

3 cups (750 mL) cherry tomatoes, halved

1 tsp (5 mL) sea salt

2 cups (500 mL) green beans, ends trimmed

2 Tbsp (30 mL) extra virgin olive oil

2 shallots, diced

1 cup (250 mL) thinly sliced button mushrooms

1 cup (250 mL) frozen corn kernels

14 oz (410 mL) can no-salt-added aduki beans, drained and rinsed

½ cup (125 mL) coarsely chopped fresh dill

2 cups (500 mL) mixed salad greens

Dressing

¼ cup (60 mL) extra virgin olive oil

2 Tbsp (30 mL) fresh lime juice

1 tsp (5 mL) balsamic vinegar

1 tsp (5 mL) Dijon mustard

¼ tsp (1 mL) sea salt

¼ tsp (1 mL) freshly ground black pepper

NUTRIENTS PER SERVING
SERVING SIZE: 1⅓ CUPS (320 ML) SALAD

238 calories, 15 g fat, 2 g saturated fat, 591 mg sodium, 23 g carbohydrates, 6 g fibre, 4 g sugars, 7 g protein. Very high in fibre. Excellent source of vitamin A, vitamin C and vitamin K. Good source of folate, magnesium and manganese.

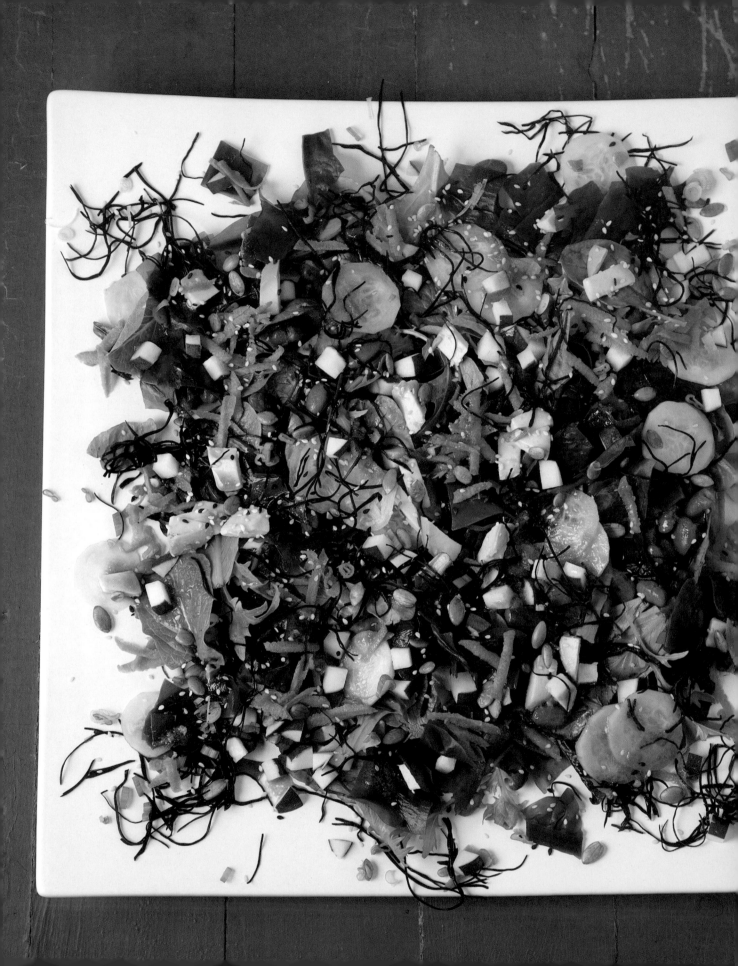

Sea Vegetable Salad with Sesame Dressing

They may be new ingredients to you, but sea vegetables (a much better name than seaweeds) like arame and wakame have been harvested from the oceans for centuries, especially in Japan. Be sure to use a bowl large enough to allow the arame and wakame to expand after it absorbs the water—they can triple in size. Sea vegetables add a briny flavour of the ocean that pairs well with wasabi, ginger and fresh lime juice. —Nettie

SERVES 6

½ cup (125 mL) dried arame sea vegetable

½ cup (125 mL) dried green wakame sea vegetable

4 cups (1 L) mixed leafy greens

14 oz (410 mL) can no-salt-added pinto beans

1 carrot, grated

4 radishes, diced

½ English cucumber, peeled and thinly sliced

1 ripe avocado, diced

1 Tbsp (15 mL) white sesame seeds, toasted

2 tsp (10 mL) black sesame seeds, toasted

1 Tbsp (15 mL) unsalted pumpkin seeds, toasted

1 green onion, thinly sliced

Dressing

2 Tbsp (30 mL) rice vinegar

2 tsp (10 mL) granulated sugar

2 tsp (10 mL) grated fresh ginger

1 tsp (5 mL) wasabi powder

2 tsp (10 mL) sodium-reduced tamari

1 Tbsp (15 mL) toasted sesame oil

2 Tbsp (30 mL) fresh lime juice

¼ tsp (1 mL) sea salt

1. Put the arame and wakame in a large bowl and cover with cold water. Let soak for 5–10 minutes until softened. Drain. Cut wakame into 1-inch (2.5 cm) pieces.

2. Place leafy greens on platter. Add arame and wakame on top of greens. Add beans. Toss.

3. To make dressing, whisk together vinegar, sugar, ginger, wasabi, tamari, sesame oil, lime juice and salt in a small bowl.

4. Spoon half the dressing over the leafy greens and sea vegetables, and toss gently. Taste and add a small amount of salt if necessary.

5. Scatter carrot, radishes, cucumber and avocado over the leafy greens. Add the remaining dressing. Sprinkle the salad with the seeds. Add green onions. Toss well and serve.

NUTRIENTS PER SERVING
SERVING SIZE: 1⅓ CUPS (320 ML) SALAD

212 calories, 10 g fat, 1 g saturated fat, 344 mg sodium, 26 g carbohydrates, 9 g fibre, 5 g sugars, 7 g protein. Very high in fibre. Excellent source of magnesium. Good source of vitamin A, vitamin C, folate, iron and zinc.

Thai Peanut Noodle Salad

If you've ever wondered how to get the authentic taste of take-out in your own kitchen, start with this recipe. It's got the wow factor; it's bursting with flavour that's so vibrant and tasty that this is sure to become a staple recipe. My kids love the peanut dressing, but I leave out the hot sauce for their "no spicy food please!" palates. —Cara

1. In a large pot of boiling water, cook linguini for 12 minutes or according to package directions. Drain and rinse with cool water. Toss noodles to keep them from sticking and set aside to drain. Transfer to a large bowl.

2. Heat oil in a large frying pan over medium-high heat. Add leeks and sauté for 3–5 minutes or until softened. Add bell peppers and sauté for another 3–5 minutes or until soft. Add carrot, edamame and cabbage. Sauté for another 3 minutes until all the vegetables are tender-crisp.

3. Remove from heat and add to drained noodles. Add cilantro and toss to combine.

4. To make the dressing, in a medium-sized bowl, whisk together peanut butter, lime zest, lime juice, oil, maple syrup, soy sauce, vinegar and hot sauce.

5. Pour over noodle mixture and stir well.

6. Add peanuts and chives and toss again.

NUTRIENTS PER SERVING
SERVING SIZE: 1⅓ CUPS (320 ML) SALAD

554 calories, 24 g fat, 4 g saturated fat, 433 mg sodium, 67 g carbohydrates, 11 g fibre, 13 g sugars, 20 g protein. Very high in fibre. Excellent source of vitamin A, vitamin C, vitamin K, thiamin, niacin, folate, manganese and iron. Good source of vitamin E, vitamin B_6 and magnesium.

SERVES 6

13 oz (375 g) whole grain linguini pasta

2 Tbsp (30 mL) extra virgin olive oil

1 leek, thinly sliced (white and pale green parts only)

1 red pepper, thinly sliced

1 yellow pepper, thinly sliced

1 carrot, grated

1½ cups (500 mL) frozen shelled edamame

¾ medium purple cabbage, thinly sliced

½ cup (125 mL) chopped fresh cilantro

Dressing

¼ cup (60 mL) smooth natural peanut butter

½ tsp (2 mL) lime zest

¼ cup (60 mL) fresh lime juice

2 Tbsp (30 mL) toasted sesame oil

1 Tbsp (15 mL) maple syrup

3 Tbsp (45 mL) sodium-reduced tamari

2 Tbsp (30 mL) balsamic vinegar

1 tsp (5 mL) hot sauce (optional)

½ cup (125 mL) roasted salted peanuts, for garnish

¼ cup (60 mL) thinly sliced fresh chives, for garnish

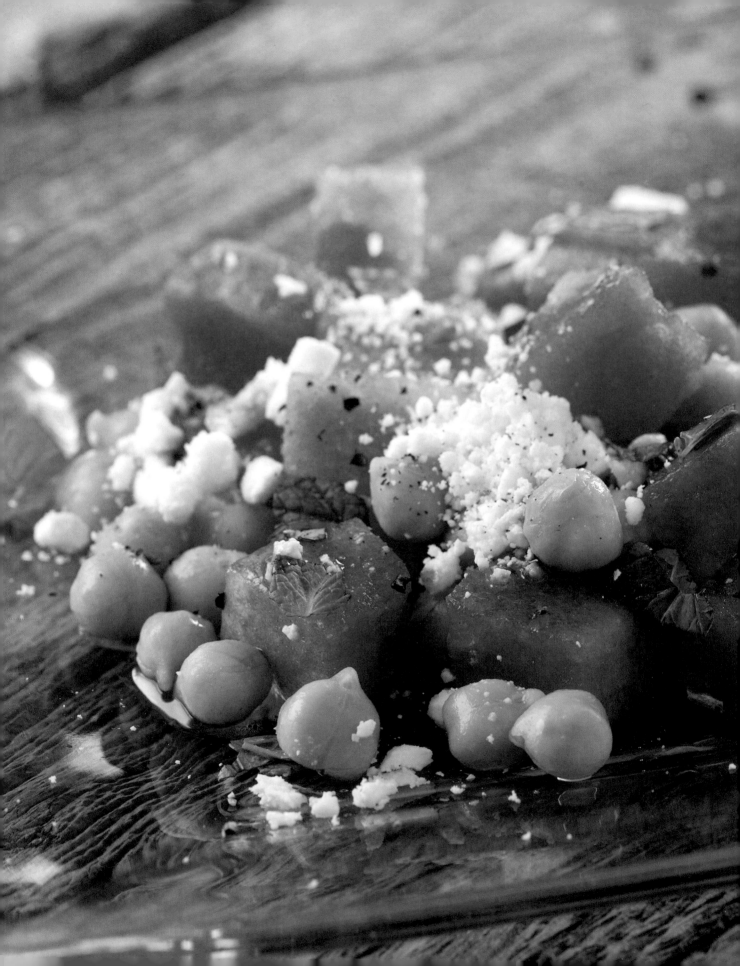

Watermelon Salad with Chickpeas, Feta & Mint

This quick and easy salad is perfect for summer barbeques. The combination of sweet watermelon, salty feta, tart balsamic vinegar and savoury mint gets all of your taste buds firing at the same time. The addition of chickpeas makes it a heartier, protein-rich option, perfect for a light lunch. —Cara

1. Arrange watermelon cubes on a large platter.

2. In a medium-sized bowl, add feta cheese and chickpeas. Stir.

3. To make dressing, in a small bowl, add pepper, oil and vinegar. Whisk to blend.

4. Pour dressing over feta cheese–chickpea mixture and toss to coat.

5. Spoon mixture on top of watermelon cubes.

6. Serve immediately, garnished with mint.

 Tip: For best results, serve this salad immediately after you prepare it. It does not store well; it gets soggy.

NUTRIENTS PER SERVING 1 CUP (250 ML) SALAD

258 calories, 16 g fat, 6 g saturated fat, 352 mg sodium, 21 g carbohydrates, 3 g fibre, 8 g sugars, 8 g protein. Excellent source of vitamin B_{12}. Good source of riboflavin, folate, calcium and zinc.

SERVES 6

4 cups (1 L) cubed seedless watermelon, removed from rind (1-inch/2.5 cm cubes)

6 oz (170 g) feta cheese, crumbled

14 oz (410 mL) can no-salt-added chickpeas, drained and rinsed

Dressing

¼ tsp (1 mL) freshly ground black pepper

¼ cup (60 mL) extra virgin olive oil

1 Tbsp (15 mL) balsamic vinegar

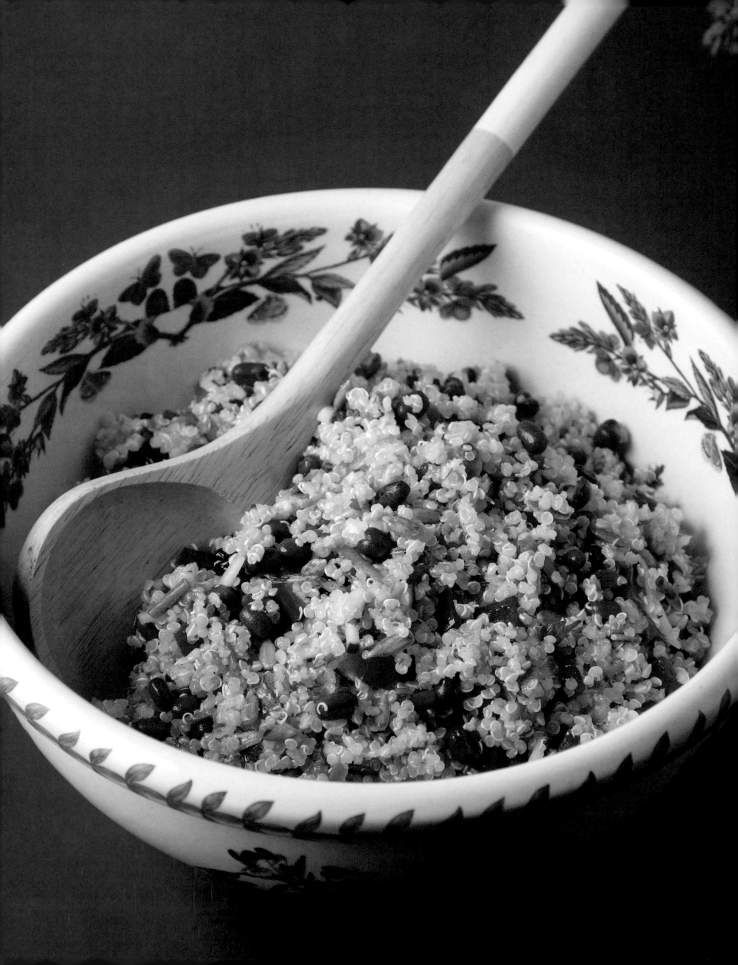

Colourful Quinoa Salad

Everyone enjoys this quinoa salad! It's got a terrific crunch from the nuts and seeds, and peppery flavour from the radishes. Plus, it's a great way to use both dried fruit and fresh vegetables. It's a full meal in a bowl! Make a double batch if you're taking it to a party—it will be a hit. —Nettie

1. Preheat the oven to 375°F (190°C).

2. Spread the seeds on a baking sheet lined with parchment paper. Toast in the oven for 8 minutes, or until golden brown. Pour them into the bowl and set aside to cool.

3. In a saucepan over high heat, bring broth, ½ tsp (2 mL) of salt and quinoa to a boil. Reduce heat to low, cover and simmer for 15 minutes, or until all of the water has been absorbed. Let stand for 5 minutes and fluff with a fork. Transfer cooked quinoa to a large bowl.

4. In a medium-sized mixing bowl, combine the lime and lemon juice, oil, cilantro, chives, and remaining ½ tsp (2 mL) salt. Whisk well. Pour on top of quinoa. Stir to combine.

5. Add the toasted seeds, aduki beans, radishes, red pepper, carrots and dried cranberries to the quinoa. Mix well and refrigerate for at least 20 minutes.

6. Taste for seasonings and add more salt if needed.

SERVES 6

⅓ cup (75 mL) raw unsalted sunflower seeds

⅓ cup (75 mL) raw unsalted pumpkin seeds

2 cups (500 mL) no-salt-added vegetable broth or water

1 tsp (5 mL) sea salt, divided

1 cup (250 mL) quinoa, rinsed

¼ cup (60 mL) fresh lime juice

¼ cup (60 mL) fresh lemon juice

⅓ cup (75 mL) extra virgin olive oil

1 cup (250 mL) chopped fresh cilantro

½ cup (125 mL) thinly sliced fresh chives

14 oz (410 mL) can no-salt-added aduki beans, drained and rinsed

4 radishes, diced

1 red pepper, diced

1 carrot, grated

½ cup (125 mL) dried cranberries

Tip: Quinoa is naturally coated with a bitter substance called saponin, which protects it from birds and critters. Rinse off the saponin to remove the bitter taste. Use a fine mesh strainer to rinse your quinoa; it will fall through the holes in a regular strainer. Hold under cold running water for 3 minutes or until there are no more bubbles and the water runs clear.

NUTRIENTS PER SERVING 1 CUP (250 ML) SALAD

400 calories, 22 g fat, 3 g saturated fat, 597 mg sodium, 42 g carbohydrates, 7 g fibre, 9 g sugars, 12 g protein. Very high in fibre. Excellent source of vitamin A, vitamin C, folate, magnesium and iron. Good source of vitamin B_6 and zinc.

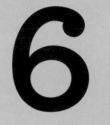

**COD & WHITE BEAN
CHOWDER, P. 102**

CHAPTER

6

Soups & Stews

Cod & White Bean Chowder

My friend Daniella and I love attending foodie events, nutrition lectures and cooking classes together—she is a dietitian too! This recipe was inspired by an exceptional chowder that we learned to make at a cooking class last year. The original version was flavoured with tarragon and saffron, had no beans and fewer vegetables. I've made it my own with some simple changes. It's easy to cook, satisfying and so very delicious. You can serve it as your main dish. —Cara

1. Heat a large pot over medium heat. Add 1 Tbsp (15 mL) olive oil. Add cod and sear each fillet for 2 minutes per side. Break it apart into bite-sized chunks. Set aside on a plate.

2. In the same pot, add remaining 1 Tbsp (15 mL) olive oil. Add shallots, celery, carrots and garlic and cook, stirring until just beginning to soften, about 5 minutes.

3. Stir in potatoes, broth, tomatoes and beans.

4. Reduce to a simmer, cover and cook until potatoes are tender, about 20 minutes.

5. Return the cod to the pot and cover. Cook until the cod is cooked through, about 4 minutes. Add salt and stir.

6. Serve garnished with fresh thyme and basil.

SERVES 6

2 Tbsp (30 mL) extra virgin olive oil, divided

1½ lb (700 g) skinless, boneless cod fillets

1 shallot, diced

2 stalks celery, diced

2 carrots, diced

2 garlic cloves, minced

1 large white potato, diced

2½ cups (625 mL) no-salt-added vegetable broth

15 oz (440 mL) can diced tomatoes and juice

14 oz (410 mL) can no-salt-added cannellini beans, drained and rinsed

½ tsp (2 mL) sea salt

1 Tbsp (15 mL) fresh thyme leaves (no stems)

1 Tbsp (15 mL) chopped fresh basil

Tip: Similar to canned beans, most cans of tomatoes have Bisphenol A (BPA) inside the lining of the can. Since the use of this chemical is questionable (see page 13), we tested recipes using tomatoes that are canned without BPA. We used Vitabio, an organic, BPA-free brand that makes crushed, diced and whole tomatoes; pasta sauce, tomato paste and even a no-salt-added product line.

NUTRIENTS PER SERVING
SERVING SIZE: 1½ CUPS (375 ML) SOUP

251 calories, 6 g fat, 1 g saturated fat, 447 mg sodium, 23 g carbohydrates, 5 g fibre, 5 g sugars, 26 g protein. High in fibre. Excellent source of vitamin A, thiamin, vitamin B_6, vitamin B_{12} and magnesium. Good source of folate.

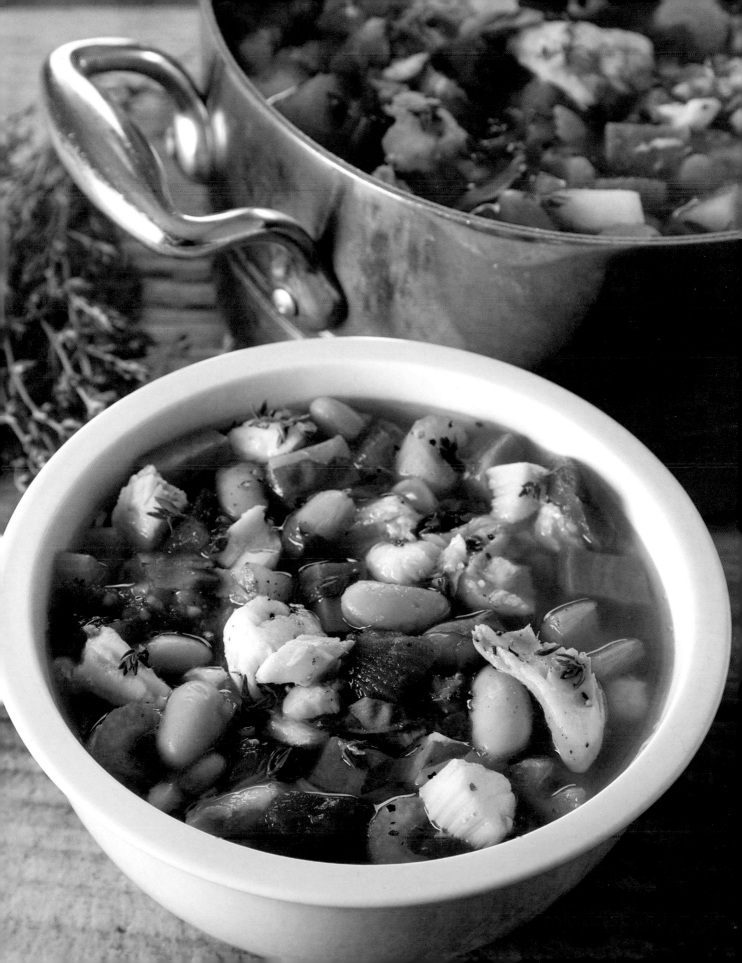

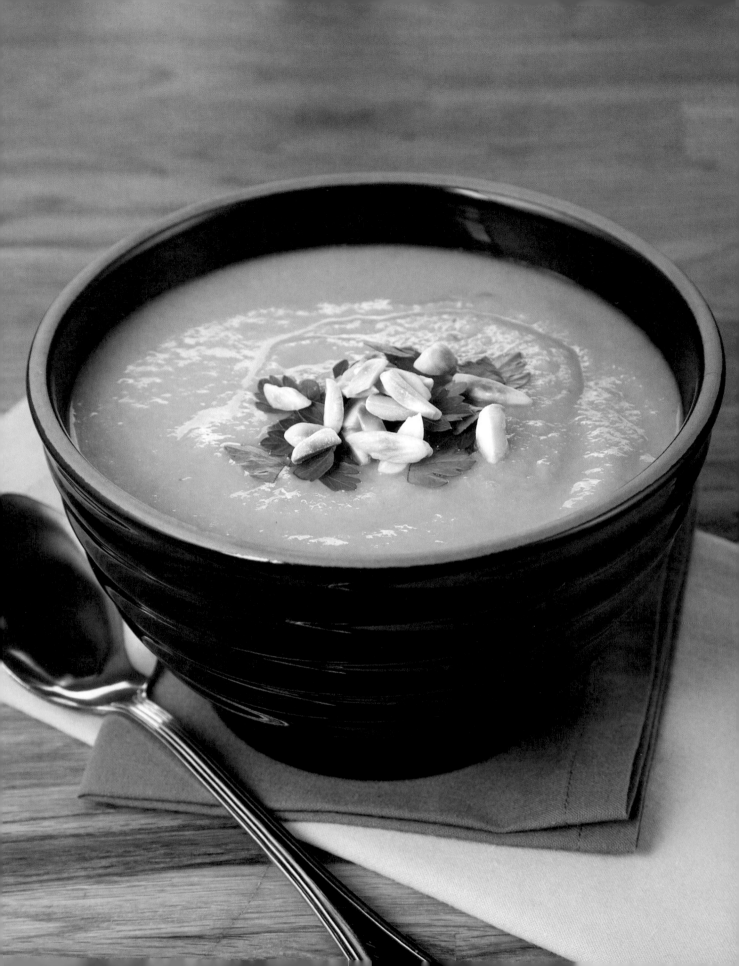

Almond, Sweet Potato & Coconut Soup

Shelled almonds are available in many forms: whole, sliced, ground and slivered. You can buy slivered almonds (cut into small wedge-shaped pieces) with their skin on or off—both work well in this soup. Additionally, adding almond butter to the soup reinforces the delicious flavour of the ingredient, and when almonds are then combined with fresh curry powder and coconut milk, it becomes a very tasty soup. —Nettie

1. Steam sweet potatoes in a steamer basket over a pot of boiling water for 10–15 minutes, or until soft when pierced with the tip of a knife.

2. In a large pot, heat olive oil over medium heat. Add onion and celery and stir, about 5 minutes. Add garlic and sauté for 1 minute.

3. Add curry powder and salt. Stir for 30 seconds.

4. Add sweet potatoes and stir well. Add broth and bring to a boil. Reduce heat and simmer for 15 minutes.

5. Remove soup from heat and cool slightly.

6. Ladle soup into a blender or food processor and blend in batches until smooth and creamy. Place soup back into saucepan on medium heat.

7. Add coconut milk, almond butter and water. Stir well to combine. Simmer soup over medium heat for 5 minutes.

8. Serve, topping with almonds and parsley.

SERVES 6

3 medium sweet potatoes, diced

1 Tbsp (15 mL) extra virgin olive oil

1 onion, diced

2 stalks celery, diced

2 garlic cloves, minced

1 tsp (5 mL) curry powder

¾ tsp (4 mL) sea salt

4 cups (1 L) no-salt-added vegetable broth

1 cup (250 mL) coconut milk

¼ cup (60 mL) almond butter

½ cup (125 mL) water

⅓ cup (75 mL) slivered almonds, toasted (see page 25)

⅓ cup (75 mL) chopped fresh parsley

NUTRIENTS PER SERVING
SERVING SIZE: 1⅔ CUPS (390 ML) SOUP

278 calories, 18 g fat, 6 g saturated fat, 364 mg sodium, 25 g carbohydrates, 4 g fibre, 9 g sugars, 6 g protein. High in fibre. Excellent source of vitamin A. Good source of magnesium.

A Note About Coconut Milk

Coconut milk is made by soaking shredded fresh coconut in hot water and squeezing out the liquid, which becomes the coconut milk. When left to stand, it separates into a layer of fatty cream and a layer of thinner milk. You can mix the two layers together with a spoon for a full-bodied flavour. Leftover coconut milk can be transferred to a resealable container and refrigerated for a maximum of 3 days.

Lily's Red Lentil Soup

When I decided to become a vegetarian at age 13, my mom, Lily, supported my decision and began experimenting with beans and lentils so I'd have something good to eat. She was a wonderful cook—and her magic with beef, chicken and fish soon found its way into her cooking with legumes too. This was the soup she'd make most often, and always to rave reviews. When I moved out to live with my boyfriend (now husband, Scott), she hand-wrote the recipe so I could take it with me. It became a weekly meal for us, and remains popular in my house to this very day. —Cara

1. In a large pot, heat oil over medium heat. Add garlic and shallot. Cook until fragrant and tender, about 3–5 minutes.

2. Add carrots, celery and sweet potato and combine well. Cook about 5 minutes.

3. Stir in red lentils and broth. Bring to a boil. Reduce heat, cover and let cook about 25 minutes, or until lentils have thickened.

4. Add dill, salt and pepper, adjusting to taste. Serve immediately.

NUTRIENTS PER SERVING
SERVING SIZE: 1⅓ CUPS (320 ML) SOUP

181 calories, 3 g fat, 0 g saturated fat, 258 mg sodium, 30 g carbohydrates, 6 g fibre, 6 g sugars, 10 g protein. Very high in fibre. Excellent source of vitamin A. Good source of iron.

SERVES 4

1 Tbsp (15 mL) extra virgin olive oil

2 garlic cloves, minced

1 shallot, minced

2 carrots, diced

1 celery stalk, diced

1 medium sweet potato, peeled and diced

1 cup (250 mL) red lentils, rinsed

4 cups (1 L) no-salt-added vegetable broth

1 tsp (5 mL) dried dill

½ tsp (2 mL) sea salt

¼ tsp (1 mL) freshly ground black pepper

Simple Vegetable Broth

You can prepare soup broth by combining a few chopped vegetables in a pot of water and simmering until the vegetables soften to release their flavour into the surrounding liquid. Soup broth can be used to add taste to sauces, stews, salad dressings, stir-fries and leafy greens. A basic broth uses onions, garlic, leeks, shallots, celery, carrots, mushrooms and tomatoes. Dominating flavours are to be avoided. That is why we do not use cabbage, broccoli, cauliflower and peppers. They overwhelm the subtle flavours of the other ingredients and can be bitter. Lentils are used to add an earthy flavour. —Nettie

1. In a large stockpot over medium heat, warm the oil. Add garlic, onion and leeks. Cook for 5 minutes, or until softened.

2. Stir in carrots and celery; cook for 8 minutes, stirring occasionally.

3. Add tomatoes, mushrooms, lentils, parsley, basil, bay leaves and pepper. Cover with water. Bring to a boil.

4. Reduce heat to low; simmer, covered, for 30 minutes, stirring often.

5. Strain through fine sieve, pressing against vegetable mixture with back of large wooden spoon to extract all the liquid. Cool before storing.

6. Store in jars in the refrigerator or freezer.

MAKES 10 CUPS (2.5 L)

2 Tbsp (30 mL) extra virgin olive oil

3 garlic cloves, minced

1 onion, diced

2 leeks, sliced thinly (white and pale green parts only)

4 carrots, diced

2 celery stalks, diced

6 medium tomatoes, quartered

3 cups (750 mL) sliced button mushrooms

⅔ cup (150 mL) green lentils

¼ cup (60 mL) chopped fresh parsley

¼ cup (60 mL) chopped fresh basil

4 bay leaves

½ tsp (2 mL) black peppercorns

10 cups (2.5 L) water

Tip: Leftover broth will keep in the fridge for 5 days. You can freeze broth in one and two cup amounts, the perfect amount for cooking many kinds of grains. Or freeze portions in ice-cube trays and use these small amounts to add flavour to stir-fries and sauces.

NUTRIENTS PER SERVING

SERVING SIZE: 1 CUP (250 ML) BROTH

8 calories, 0 g fat, 0 g saturated fat, 60 mg sodium, 2 g carbohydrates, 0 g fibre, 0 g sugars, 0 g protein.

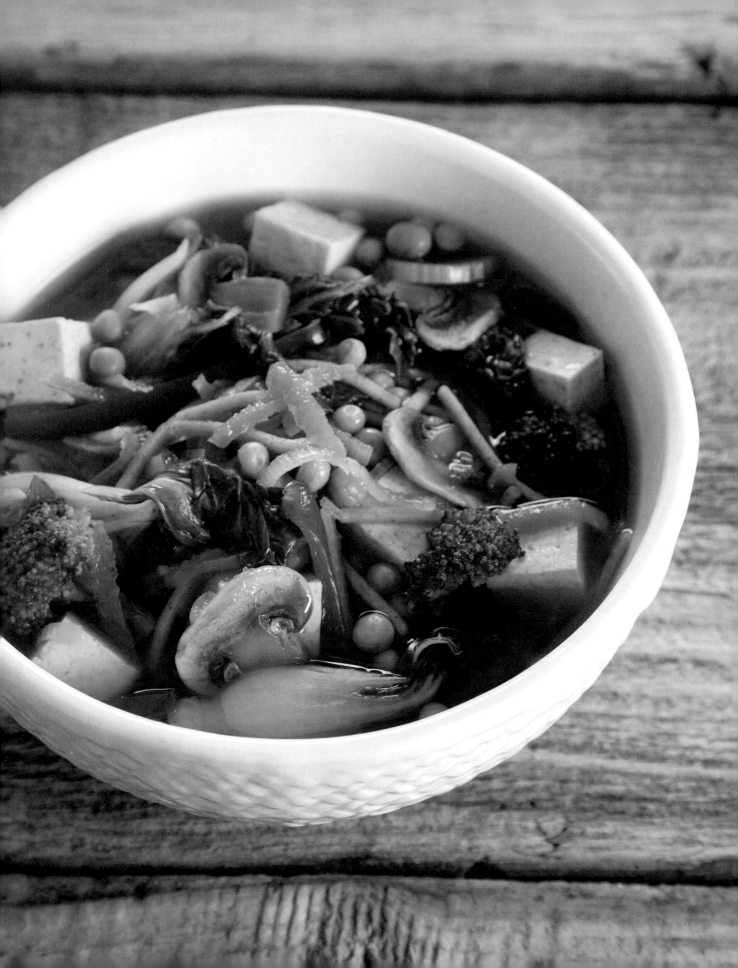

Asian Vegetable Noodle Soup

Colourful and hearty, this soup is surprisingly simple to make. When I travel for business, this is my husband, Scott's, go-to recipe to make for the kids. I eat the leftovers when I get home! —Cara

1. In a large pot, bring 1 cup (250 mL) vegetable broth to a boil. Add leek, garlic and ginger, and simmer for 3 minutes. Stir in remaining broth, tamari, miso and kombu. Cover and bring to a boil for about 10 minutes. Remove kombu.

2. Add carrot, celery, bok choy, broccoli, red pepper, mushrooms, peas, noodles and tofu. Simmer for about 10 minutes, or until noodles are softened. Serve.

A Note About Umami

Have you heard of *umami*? It's considered to be the fifth taste, after salty, sour, bitter and sweet. It's best described as "savoury," and one great way to get this flavour is to add seaweed to your foods. Kombu has that unique *umami* flavour, and using more *umami*-rich foods (tomatoes, Parmesan cheese and mushrooms also have it), can reduce your reliance on salt in many recipes.

NUTRIENTS PER SERVING
SERVING SIZE: 1⅓ CUPS (320 ML) SOUP

209 calories, 6 g fat, 1 g saturated fat, 498 mg sodium, 27 g carbohydrates, 3 g fibre, 9 g sugars, 14 g protein. Excellent source of vitamin C. Good source of folate, magnesium and iron.

SERVES 6

6 cups (1.5 L) no-salt-added vegetable broth, divided

1 leek, thinly sliced (white and pale green parts only)

2 garlic cloves, minced

1 Tbsp (15 mL) minced ginger

2 Tbsp (30 mL) sodium-reduced tamari

2 tsp (10 mL) white miso paste

Two 4-inch (10 cm) squares of kombu

1 carrot, grated

1 stalk celery, thinly sliced

3 stalks bok choy, diagonally sliced

1 cup (250 mL) broccoli florets

1 red pepper, julienned

1 cup (250 mL) thinly sliced mushrooms

½ cup (125 mL) peas (fresh or frozen)

3 oz (90 g) buckwheat soba noodles, broken into 1-inch (2.5 cm) pieces (about ¾ cup/ 175 mL)

12 oz (350 g) tofu, cubed (½ inch/1 cm)

Pinto Bean & Brown Rice Soup with Apricots

This recipe has one of my favourite blends of spices. Combining the earthy flavour of cinnamon with the sweet taste of cardamom, the heat of cayenne and the full flavour of paprika allows each ingredient to shine. The dried spices I use are from Peter Piper Pepper, a Canadian company that sells Organic Fair Trade spices in small resealable pouches. The apricots are a unique treasure to find in this hearty soup—they're not your everyday soup bowl ingredient. They make this soup extra special. —Nettie

1. In a medium-sized saucepan, bring 2 cups (500 mL) of broth to a boil over high heat. Stir in rice. Cover, reduce heat and simmer for 45–50 minutes, or until rice is tender.

2. In a large skillet over medium-high heat, heat oil. Add onion, zucchini and red pepper. Cook for 5 minutes or until just softened. Add beans.

3. Add tomatoes, cinnamon, cardamom, cayenne, paprika and salt. Cover, reduce heat to low and cook for 8 minutes or until tender.

4. In a large pot, bring remaining 8 cups (2 L) broth to a boil. Reduce heat to a simmer and add apricots. Simmer for 10 minutes, covered.

5. Stir vegetables and cooked rice into large pot and simmer for 10 minutes to desired consistency.

6. Serve, sprinkled with basil.

 Tip: This make a very large pot of soup on purpose—freeze the leftovers for a quick and easy meal another night.

SERVES 8

10 cups (2.5 L) no-salt-added vegetable broth, divided

1 cup (250 mL) short-grain brown rice

2 Tbsp (30 mL) extra virgin olive oil

1 onion, diced

1 zucchini, thinly sliced

1 red pepper, diced

14 oz (410 mL) can no-salt-added pinto beans, drained

2 medium tomatoes, diced

½ tsp (2 mL) ground cinnamon

¼ tsp (1 mL) ground cardamom

¼ tsp (1 mL) cayenne

1 Tbsp (15 mL) paprika

1 tsp (5 mL) sea salt

1 cup (250 mL) dried apricots, chopped

2 Tbsp (30 mL) chopped fresh basil

NUTRIENTS PER SERVING
SERVING SIZE: 1½ CUPS (375 ML) SOUP

220 calories, 4 g fat, 1 g saturated fat, 305 mg sodium, 42 g carbohydrates, 5 g fibre, 16 g sugars, 6 g protein. High in fibre. Good source of vitamin C.

Mango, Carrot & Parsnip Soup

This creamy soul-warming soup is the perfect autumn comfort food. Look for firm, medium-sized parsnips with smooth surfaces; large ones are often split, with bitter, woody inner cores. Sweet, buttery parsnips remind me of cream-coloured carrots and pair perfectly with mango in this recipe. —Nettie

1. In a large pot, heat oil over medium heat. Sauté leeks and garlic in oil for 3–5 minutes or until softened.

2. Add parsnips, carrots and mango. Stir. Add broth. Simmer, covered, over low heat for 30 minutes. Stir often.

3. Transfer in batches to food processor or blender. Process until smooth.

4. Return to pot over medium heat. Add salt, pepper and nutmeg. Stir.

5. Whisk in soy beverage, if using.

6. Serve and garnish individual bowls with toasted pumpkin seeds.

Tip: With the arrival of winter, having frozen fruit on hand is always a smart idea. It's affordable, saves time and often comes in resealable pouches. With frozen fruit, there's no need to wait for it to ripen, and no waste of over-ripe fruit!

NUTRIENTS PER SERVING
SERVING SIZE: 1⅓ CUPS (320 ML) SOUP

260 calories, 14 g fat, 2 g saturated fat, 150 mg sodium, 31 g carbohydrates, 6 g fibre, 17 g sugars, 8 g protein. Very high in fibre. Excellent source of folate and magnesium. Good source of vitamin A, vitamin C, iron and zinc.

SERVES 6

2 Tbsp (30 mL) extra virgin olive oil

2 leeks, diced (white and pale green parts only)

3 garlic cloves, minced

4 medium parsnips, peeled and sliced into rounds

2 carrots, sliced into rounds

2 cups (500 mL) frozen cubed mango pieces (½ inch/1 cm)

6 cups (1.5 L) no-salt-added vegetable broth

¼ tsp (1 mL) sea salt

¼ tsp (1 mL) freshly ground black pepper

¼ tsp (1 mL) ground nutmeg

1 cup (250 mL) plain fortified soy beverage (optional)

½ cup (125 mL) unsalted pumpkin seeds, toasted (see page 25), for garnish

Tofu Minestrone

Tofu can be easily crumbled, and it does a fantastic job of absorbing the flavours of your soup broth. We use 12 cups of stock in this recipe because we cook the pasta in the pot, and it absorbs lots of liquid as it cooks. You can use an assortment of different greens in this soup—we used kale, but spinach, chard or collards would work equally well. —Nettie

1. In large pot, heat 1 cup (250 mL) of the broth over medium heat. Add leeks and cook for 5 minutes or until softened.

2. Add garlic, carrot, celery, tomatoes, basil, oregano and remaining broth; bring to boil. Reduce heat and simmer until vegetables are tender, about 10 minutes.

3. Add pasta; cook until tender, 10–12 minutes or according to package directions.

4. Stir in tofu, beans, basil, salt, cayenne and kale. Simmer for 5 minutes.

5. Serve and sprinkle each serving with Asiago cheese.

 Tip: Asiago is a strong-flavoured hard cheese, similar to Parmesan or Romano. You can use any of them interchangeably in this recipe.

NUTRIENTS PER SERVING
SERVING SIZE: 1¾ CUPS (425 ML) SOUP

221 calories, 6 g fat, 2 g saturated fat, 500 mg sodium, 33 g carbohydrates, 6 g fibre, 8 g sugars, 13 g protein. Very high in fibre. Good source of vitamin A, folate, vitamin C, calcium and iron.

SERVES 8

12 cups (3 L) no-salt-added vegetable broth or water, divided

1 leek, diced (white and pale green parts only)

3 garlic cloves, minced

1 carrot, grated

2 stalks celery, thinly sliced

28 oz (795 mL) can crushed tomatoes

2 tsp (10 mL) dried basil

2 tsp (10 mL) dried oregano

1 cup (250 mL) whole grain rotini

½ lb (225 g) firm tofu, crumbled

14 oz (410 mL) can no-salt-added aduki beans, drained and rinsed

¼ cup (60 mL) chopped fresh basil

¾ tsp (4 mL) sea salt

¼ tsp (1 mL) cayenne pepper

2 cups (500 mL) baby kale, chopped

½ cup (125 mL) grated Asiago cheese

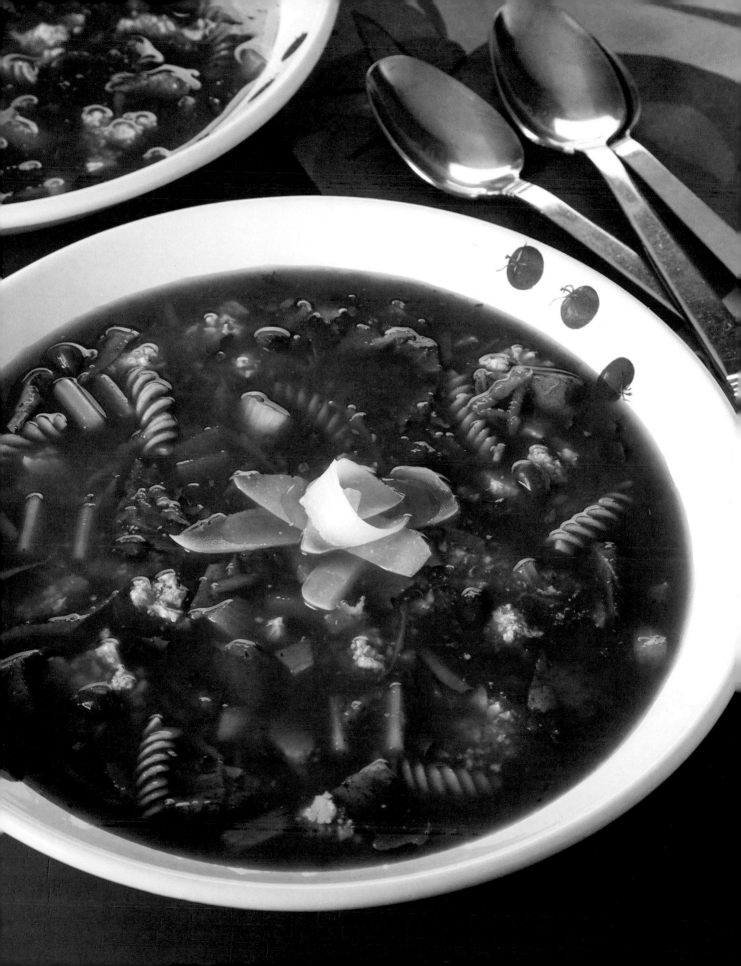

Tip: Tomatillos look like small green tomatoes but have a papery covering. They are in the tomato family but are unique due to their distinctive tart flavour. If you can't find tomatillos, buy four under-ripe tomatoes and add a teaspoon of lime juice.

Tortilla & Tomatillo Soup with Lime-Chia Yogurt

This soup quickly became our favourite on the day we tested it, and our families agreed when they tasted the leftovers. The pronounced flavour of corn tortillas is such a welcome surprise in a creamy soup, and the spiciness from the ancho chili powder is cooled by the thick lime-chia yogurt on top. —Cara

1. Under a broiler, dry roast the tomato, tomatillo, red pepper and jalapeno until charred. Set aside to cool, about 5 minutes.

2. Peel and seed the red pepper and jalapeno. Coarsely chop the charred vegetables.

3. In a medium-sized pot over medium heat, add 2 Tbsp (30 mL) of the olive oil, shallot and garlic, stirring occasionally for a few minutes. Add chopped roasted vegetables, ancho chili powder, salt and pepper.

4. Add broth, bring to boil, cover, reduce heat and simmer for 25 minutes.

5. Meanwhile, in a skillet, add 1 tsp (5 mL) of the oil and brown corn tortillas for about 1 minute on each side, adding remaining oil as needed. Let tortillas cool. Break into pieces.

6. Pour about half of the soup into a blender or use an immersion blender in the pot. Add half of the tortillas and purée until smooth. Repeat with remaining soup and tortillas.

7. To make the chia-lime yogurt, in a medium bowl, whisk together Greek yogurt, lime juice and chia seeds. Set aside for 10 minutes to allow flavours to combine and yogurt to thicken.

8. To serve, pour soup into bowls and garnish with yogurt mixture, cilantro and a squeeze of lime to taste.

NUTRIENTS PER SERVING
SERVING SIZE: 1⅓ CUPS (320 ML) SOUP
PLUS ⅙ CHIA-LIME YOGURT

170 calories, 9 g fat, 2 g saturated fat, 238 mg sodium, 19 g carbohydrates, 4 g fibre, 8 g sugars, 6 g protein. High in fibre. Excellent source of vitamin C.

SERVES 6

4 large tomatoes

8 tomatillos

1 red pepper

1 jalapeno pepper

3 Tbsp (45 mL) extra virgin olive oil, divided

1 shallot, diced

4 garlic cloves, minced

1 tsp (5 mL) ancho chili powder

½ tsp (2 mL) sea salt

¼ tsp (1 mL) freshly ground black pepper

2 cups (500 mL) no-salt-added vegetable broth

4 corn tortillas (4 inch/10 cm)

½ cup (125 mL) chopped fresh cilantro

2 limes

Lime-Chia Yogurt

1 cup (250 mL) 2% Greek yogurt

¼ cup (60 mL) fresh lime juice

1 Tbsp (15 mL) chia seeds

Roasted Tomato & Lentil Soup with Steel-Cut Oats

You may have rolled oats on hand, but don't be tempted to use them in place of steel-cut oats in this recipe; they are not the same ingredient. Steel-cut oats are the oval-shaped whole oat groat, which is cut into several pieces by a sharp steel roller. They retain a toothsome chew when cooked, and they never lose their shape entirely. Rolled oats are steamed, then pressed between rollers and dried. The result cooks quicker than steel-cut oats and does not retain the texture that this soup requires. —Cara

1. Preheat oven to 425°F (220°C).
2. Drain the canned tomatoes in a colander set over a bowl. Using your hands, gently break open the tomatoes allowing more juice to drain into the bowls. Reserve the juices.
3. Line a baking sheet with aluminum foil and arrange tomatoes in a single layer. Drizzle with 2 Tbsp (30 mL) of the olive oil. Sprinkle with salt, pepper and sugar. Roast for 20 minutes.
4. Add garlic cloves and roast another 10 minutes. In a separate bowl, coarsely mash and set aside.
5. In a large saucepan, sauté onions in remaining olive oil until cooked through.
6. Into the saucepan, add the reserved tomato juice, broth, lentils, oats, tomato paste, sun-dried tomatoes, oregano, basil and roasted tomato mixture.
7. Bring to boil, reduce heat and simmer, stirring often, for 25 minutes, until lentils are tender.
8. Serve hot in soup bowls.

NUTRIENTS PER SERVING
SERVING SIZE: 1¼ CUPS (300 ML)

238 calories, 6 g fat, 1 g saturated fat, 500 mg sodium, 38 g carbohydrates, 7 g fibre, 15 g sugars, 10 g protein. Very high in fibre. Excellent source of vitamin C. Good source of iron.

SERVES 8

2 cans (28 oz/830 mL) whole plum tomatoes

3 Tbsp (45 mL) extra virgin olive oil, divided

½ tsp (2 mL) sea salt

¼ tsp (1 mL) freshly ground black pepper

1 Tbsp (15 mL) brown sugar

4 garlic cloves, peeled

1 red onion, diced

8 cups (2 L) no-salt-added vegetable broth

1 cup (250 mL) red lentils, drained and rinsed

⅓ cup (75 mL) steel-cut oats

¼ cup (60 mL) tomato paste

2 Tbsp (30 mL) finely chopped sun-dried tomatoes

1 tsp (5 mL) dried oregano

1 tsp (5 mL) dried basil

African Peanut Soup

On recipe testing days, I'd call my dad at the office and let him know what was on the menu. He'd stop by on his way home from work to sample a bit of everything. He's my favourite recipe taster because he loves a wide range of foods, isn't afraid to be honest and gives the best feedback. Thanks, Dad! This soup was his absolute favourite. He liked the complex flavour profile, the subtle spice and the fact that he'd never tasted anything quite like it before. —Cara

1. In large saucepan, heat the olive oil over medium heat. Sauté the ginger and garlic for 1–2 minutes, or until soft and fragrant.

2. Add onion and sweet potato and sauté for about 5 minutes, or until the onion is softened. Stir in cumin and red pepper flakes.

3. Add the tomato paste and peanut butter, and stir until everything is evenly mixed. Add the vegetable broth and stir to dissolve the thick tomato paste–peanut butter mixture.

4. Bring to boil, reduce heat to low and simmer 15–20 minutes, or until the sweet potatoes are soft. Once soft, mash about half of the sweet potatoes to help thicken the soup.

5. Add spinach and cook another 2–3 minutes, or until spinach wilts.

6. Serve garnished with cilantro and peanuts.

NUTRIENTS PER SERVING
SERVING SIZE: 1⅓ CUPS (320 ML) SOUP

305 calories, 19 g fat, 3 g saturated fat, 141 mg sodium, 26 g carbohydrates, 6 g fibre, 12 g sugars, 11 g protein. Very high in fibre. Excellent source of vitamin A and folate. Good source of magnesium and iron.

SERVES 6

1 Tbsp (15 mL) extra virgin olive oil

1 Tbsp (15 mL) fresh ginger, grated

3 garlic cloves, minced

1 red onion, diced

1 medium sweet potato, peeled and diced

1 tsp (5 mL) ground cumin

¼ tsp (1 mL) crushed red pepper flakes

5 oz (150 mL) can tomato paste

½ cup (125 mL) natural chunky peanut butter

6 cups (1.5 L) no-salt-added vegetable broth

4 cups (1 L) spinach, cut into strips

¼ cup (60 mL) chopped fresh cilantro, for garnish

½ cup (125 mL) unsalted roasted peanuts, for garnish

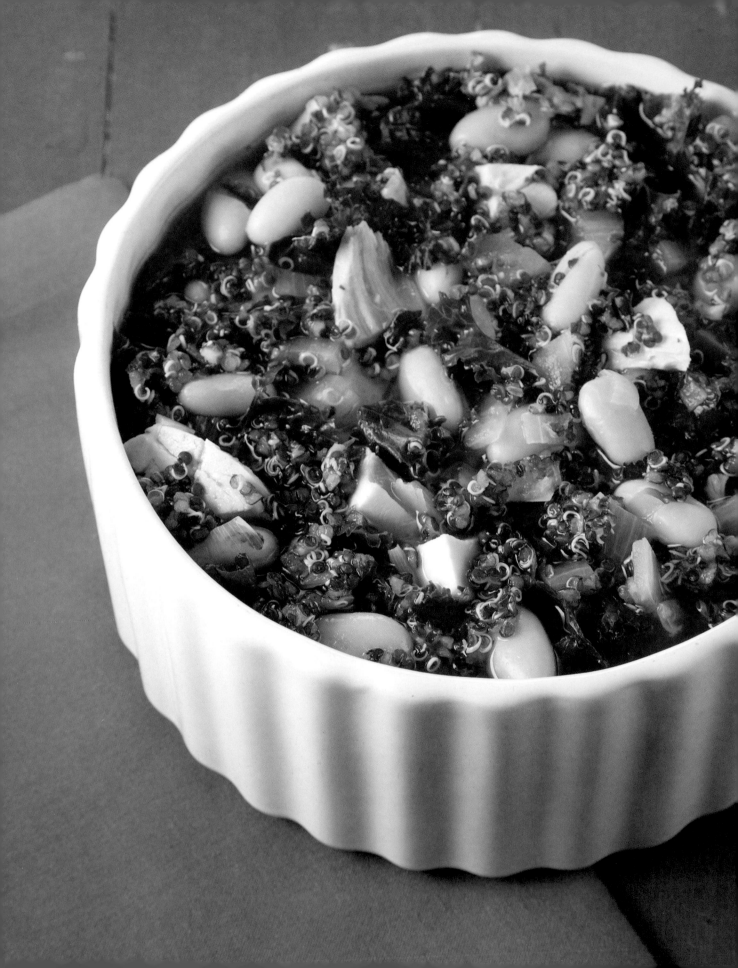

Chicken, Beans & Greens Stew

This warming stew is a modern take on traditional chicken soup with rice. The red quinoa adds beautiful colour and texture, and using the pre-cooked chicken allows you to cook this soup in about 25 minutes. It's a quick and delicious weeknight meal, and the leftovers make a great lunch. We served this as lunch to the photography and food styling team for this book on one of the photoshoot days, and we were met with very enthusiastic thumbs-up. —Cara

1. In a large pot over high heat, combine the broth, onion, quinoa, oregano, garlic and bay leaf. Bring to a boil. Reduce to a simmer, cover and cook for 20–25 minutes.

2. Remove lid and add kidney beans and kale. Cook until the kale has wilted, about 3 minutes.

3. Stir in the chicken, season with salt and pepper, remove bay leaf and serve.

Tip: If you can't find red quinoa, you can use tan quinoa too. However, be sure to reduce the cooking time in step 1 to just 15 minutes rather than 20 minutes, since tan quinoa cooks faster than red quinoa.

NUTRIENTS PER SERVING
SERVING SIZE: 2 CUPS (500 ML) STEW

221 calories, 5 g fat, 1 g saturated fat, 434 mg sodium, 24 g carbohydrates, 5 g fibre, 3 g sugars, 21 g protein. High in fibre. Excellent source of vitamin A and thiamin. Good source of niacin and vitamin C.

SERVES 4

6 cups (1.5 L) no-salt-added chicken broth

1 onion, diced

½ cup (125 mL) red quinoa, rinsed

1½ tsp (2 mL) dried oregano

1 garlic clove, minced

1 bay leaf

14 oz (410 mL) can no-salt-added white kidney beans, drained and rinsed

2 cups (500 mL) chopped kale

2 cups (500 mL) diced cooked rotisserie chicken

¼ tsp (1 mL) freshly ground black pepper

¼ tsp (1 mL) sea salt

Vegetable Soup with Pistou

Pistou is similar to the well-known Italian pesto, but this French version doesn't contain pine nuts. We added pumpkin seeds to our version for a depth of flavour and a touch of whimsy. After the soup has simmered to perfection, a dollop of pistou is added to each bowl and gently swirled in. The herbs from the pistou diffuse into the soup, transforming the broth into a magical elixir that's filled with flavour. This soup has it all; it is aromatic, tasty and visually appealing too! Store leftovers with pistou mixed in to infuse the flavour. —Cara

SERVES 8

2 Tbsp (30 mL) extra virgin olive oil

2 shallots, diced

2 carrots, diced

1 leek, diced (white and pale green parts only)

1 small fennel bulb, diced

1 celery stalk, diced

4 cups (1 L) no-salt-added vegetable broth

3 plum tomatoes, seeded and finely diced

4 cups (1 L) water

½ cup (125 mL) green beans cut into 1-inch (2.5 cm) lengths

¼ cup (60 mL) whole grain fusilli

14 oz (410 mL) can no-salt-added pinto beans, drained and rinsed

¼ tsp (1 mL) sea salt, or more to taste

⅛ tsp (0.5 mL) freshly ground black pepper

Pistou

½ cup (125 mL) extra virgin olive oil, divided

½ cup (125 mL) raw unsalted pumpkin seeds

2 garlic cloves, minced

2 cups (500 mL) chopped fresh parsley

½ cup (125 mL) fresh basil

½ cup (125 mL) grated Parmesan cheese

½ tsp (2 mL) sea salt

¼ tsp (1 mL) freshly ground black pepper

1. In a large saucepan, heat the olive oil over medium heat. Add shallots and cook until translucent, about 8 minutes.

2. Add the carrots, leek, fennel and celery. Cook until softened, about 6 minutes.

3. Add the broth, tomatoes and water. Bring to a boil. Reduce the heat, cover partially and simmer until vegetables are tender, about 15 minutes.

4. Add the green beans, fusilli and beans and cook about 10–12 minutes until pasta is cooked. Season with salt and pepper.

5. For the pistou, in a small skillet, heat ¼ cup (60 mL) olive oil. Add the pumpkin seeds and garlic and cook over medium heat until the seeds turn light brown, about 3 minutes. Scrape the contents of the skillet into a food processor. Add the parsley, basil, Parmesan, salt, pepper and remaining ¼ cup (60 mL) olive oil and process until smooth.

6. To serve, ladle soup into bowls. Add a tablespoon of pistou to each bowl and gently swirl it into the soup.

NUTRIENTS PER SERVING

SERVING SIZE: 1¼ CUPS (300 ML) SOUP PLUS 1 TBSP (15 ML) PISTOU

232 calories, 14 g fat, 2 g saturated fat, 325 mg sodium, 22 g carbohydrates, 6 g fibre, 5 g sugars, 7 g protein. Very high in fibre. Excellent source of magnesium. Good source of vitamin A, folate, vitamin C and iron.

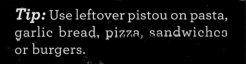

Tip: Use leftover pistou on pasta, garlic bread, pizza, sandwiches or burgers.

Hearty Veggie Stew

Pots of stew and chili taste better the second day.
I recommend preparing this recipe ahead of time. My
daughter Macko and I cook large batches of stew and
freeze it for upcoming dinners or events. It can also be
kept warm all day in a slow cooker without drying out.
You can make this as spicy as you like by adjusting the
amount of chili powder you use. —Nettie

1. In a large skillet, heat the oil over medium heat. Add the
   onions and cook, stirring until lightly browned, about 3–5
   minutes. Add the mushrooms and celery and continue cooking
   for 5 minutes.
2. Reduce heat to medium, stir in cumin, oregano, chili powder
   and garlic. Add zucchini, tomatoes, tomato paste, sun-dried
   tomatoes, tofu and broth. Stir well. Cook for 5 minutes.
3. Add beans, corn, salt and pepper. Reduce heat to low, cover
   and simmer for 15 minutes, stirring occasionally.
4. Serve garnished with cheddar, cilantro and cashews.

Tip: Don't add the cashews if you are going
to freeze the stew. They change colour and do
not look as appetizing as they could. Add them
when you defrost the stew.

NUTRIENTS PER SERVING
SERVING SIZE: 1⅔ CUPS (390 ML) STEW

418 calories, 23 g fat, 7 g saturated fat, 311 mg sodium, 34 g
carbohydrates, 8 g fibre, 11 g sugars, 23 g protein. Very high in fibre.
Excellent source of folate, calcium, magnesium, iron and zinc.
Good source of riboflavin, vitamin B₆ and vitamin C.

SERVES 6

2 Tbsp (30 mL) extra virgin olive oil

2 Vidalia or other sweet onions, diced

1 cup (250 mL) chopped mushrooms

2 stalks celery, diced

1 Tbsp (15 mL) ground cumin

1 tsp (5 mL) dry oregano

2 tsp (10 mL) chili powder

4 garlic cloves, minced

1 medium zucchini, diced

2 large tomatoes, diced

¼ cup (60 mL) tomato paste

¼ cup (60 mL) diced sun-dried tomatoes

12 oz (350 g) firm tofu, crumbled

2 cups (500 mL) no-salt-added vegetable broth

14 oz (410 mL) can no-salt-added black beans, drained

1 cup (250 mL) frozen corn kernels

¼ tsp (1 mL) kosher salt

⅛ tsp (0.5 mL) freshly ground black pepper

1 cup (250 mL) grated cheddar cheese

⅓ cup (75 mL) chopped fresh cilantro leaves

½ cup (125 mL) toasted cashews (see toasting instructions, page 25)

White Bean Rosemary Soup with Garlic Croutons

The garlicky croutons are the key to this mild-tasting, smooth soup. Use a good-quality whole grain or sprouted bread, such as the loaves made by Stonemill Bakehouse. Artisan or sprouted breads that are slowly fermented, rather than those made with quick-rising yeast, tend to be easier to digest. Croutons are best when made with day-old bread. —Cara

SERVES 6

Croutons

3 slices whole grain bread, preferably day-old

2 Tbsp (30 mL) extra virgin olive oil

1 tsp (5 mL) garlic powder

2 Tbsp (30 mL) grated Parmesan cheese

Soup

1 Tbsp (15 mL) extra virgin olive oil

4 garlic cloves, minced

1 onion, diced

2 carrots, cut into coins

2 stalks celery, sliced

4 cups (1 L) no-salt-added vegetable broth

2 cans (14 oz/410 mL each) no-salt-added cannellini beans, drained and rinsed

2 Tbsp (30 mL) chopped fresh rosemary

½ tsp (2 mL) sea salt

¼ tsp (1 mL) freshly ground black pepper

1. To make croutons, preheat oven to 350°F (180°C). Cut bread into medium bite-sized cubes. Add cubes to a medium bowl and toss with olive oil, garlic powder and Parmesan. Spread cubes on a baking sheet lined with parchment paper and bake for 15 minutes or until crisp. Turn halfway to ensure even baking.

2. In a large saucepan, heat oil over medium heat. Add garlic, onion, carrots and celery and cook for about 5 minutes. Add broth and bring to a boil; reduce heat and cook for 20 minutes, carrots should be very tender.

3. Add beans and rosemary; cook 10 more minutes.

4. With an immersion blender or in a blender, purée the soup until smooth. Season with salt and pepper. Set aside.

5. Serve soup topped with croutons.

NUTRIENTS PER SERVING SERVING SIZE: 1⅓ CUPS (320 ML) SOUP WITH CROUTONS

205 calories, 7 g fat, 1 g saturated fat, 359 mg sodium, 30 g carbohydrates, 7 g fibre, 5 g sugars, 8 g protein. Very high in fibre. Excellent source of thiamin. Good source of vitamin A.

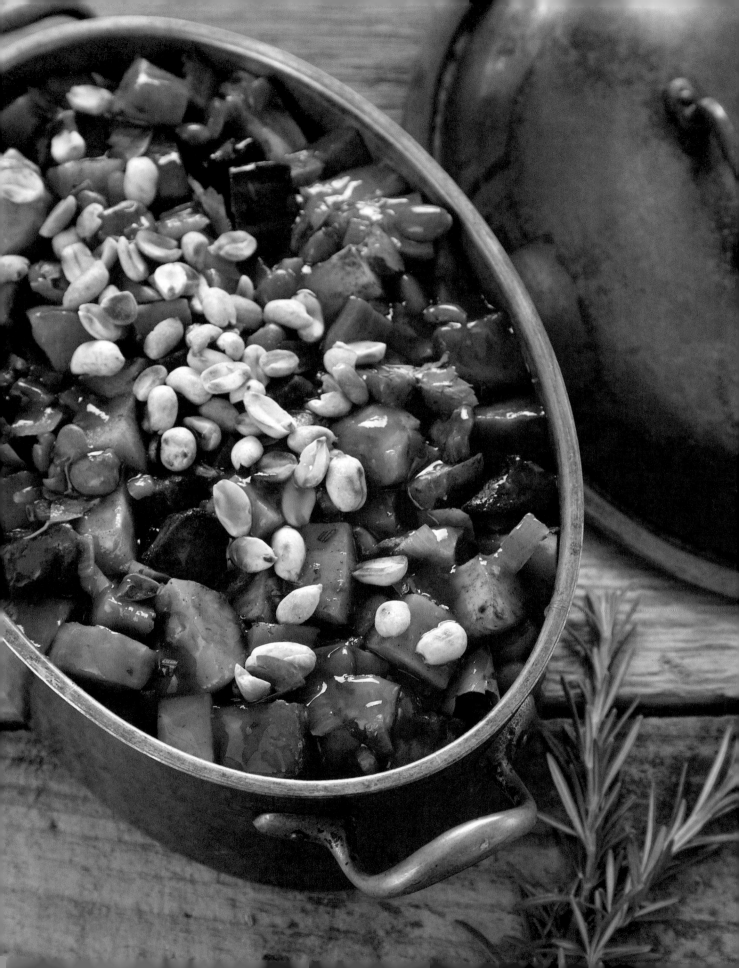

Underground Stew

The common theme in this stew is that it is based on the goodness from under the earth. Peanuts, carrots, celery root, sweet potatoes and parsnip all grow underground and retain a rich array of vitamins and minerals from the soil. We roasted vegetables in the oven with a small amount of oil to coat them and seal in their moisture. The dry heat intensifies the flavours of vegetables, leaving them tender on the inside and crispy on the outside. —Nettie

1. Preheat oven to 400°F (200°C). Line a rimmed baking sheet with parchment paper.

2. In a large bowl mix carrots, celery root, parsnips and sweet potatoes with ¼ cup (60 mL) olive oil, ½ tsp (2 mL) salt, pepper, cinnamon, paprika and nutmeg. Transfer to baking sheet in a single layer and roast until they are fork-tender, about 25 minutes.

3. Heat the remaining 1 Tbsp (15 mL) oil in a large stockpot over medium heat. Add onions and allow to brown, 3–5 minutes, stirring occasionally to prevent burning.

4. Add wine and cook until it is reduced by half, 3–5 minutes.

5. Add broth and beans and bring to a boil. Add the roasted vegetables. Reduce heat and simmer, stirring occasionally, for 15 minutes.

6. Add rosemary and parsley to the stew, remove from heat. Add to serving bowls and garnish with peanuts.

NUTRIENTS PER SERVING
SERVING SIZE: 1⅔ CUPS (390 ML) STEW

328 calories, 16 g fat, 2 g saturated fat, 500 mg sodium, 39 g carbohydrates, 9 g fibre, 12 g sugars, 7 g protein. Very high in fibre. Excellent source of vitamin A and folate. Good source of magnesium and iron.

SERVES 6

4 carrots, diced

1 celery root, diced

2 parsnips, diced

1 medium sweet potato, peeled and diced

¼ cup (60 mL) plus 1 Tbsp (15 mL) extra virgin olive oil, divided

1 tsp (5 mL) sea salt, divided

¼ tsp (1 mL) freshly ground pepper

1 tsp (5 mL) ground cinnamon

1 tsp (5 mL) paprika

¼ tsp (1 mL) ground nutmeg

1 onion, diced

½ cup (125 mL) dry white wine

4 cups (1 L) no-salt-added vegetable broth

14 oz (410 mL) no-salt-added pinto beans, drained and rinsed

2 tsp (10 mL) finely chopped fresh rosemary

2 tsp (10 mL) finely chopped fresh flat-leaf parsley

¼ cup (60 mL) roasted, salted peanuts, for garnish

A Note About Salt

SODIUM IN THE DIET—WHERE DOES IT COME FROM?

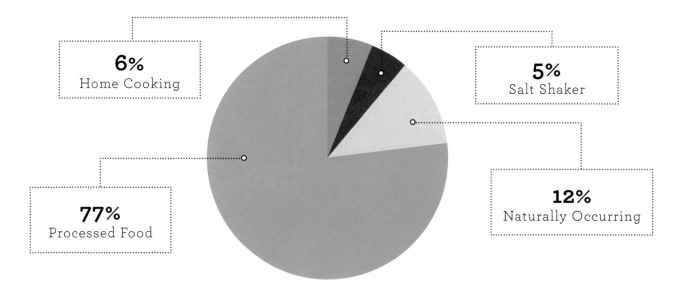

6%
Home Cooking

5%
Salt Shaker

77%
Processed Food

12%
Naturally Occurring

Canadians like salty food, and our personal sodium intake can be quite high if we rely heavily on processed foods. About 77 percent of the sodium we eat comes from processed foods and restaurant meals. Only 6 percent comes from the meals we cook at home, which means that cooking from scratch more often helps reduce your sodium intake.

While a small amount of sodium is required for normal muscle functioning, most Canadians consume double the amount that they need. The average Canadian gets a whopping 3,400 mg/day of sodium, which far exceeds the recommended intake of just 1,500 mg/day.

When we think of sodium, we may think about that salt shaker on the table, but that sprinkle of salt we add at the table accounts for just 5 percent of the sodium in the diet. Sodium is widely used as a preservative, not just as a flavour enhancer. That means foods that don't taste salty, such as candy or pre-sweetened breakfast cereal, may be really high in salt in a form of a sodium-based preservative.

READ LABELS

When grocery shopping, it's a good idea to compare nutrition tables on different brands and see where you can cut back on sodium. It's important because excess salt can lead to hypertension (high blood pressure), which is a major cause of heart disease. It's is also a risk factor for stroke and kidney disease.

If you do need to cut back on salt, eliminating high-sodium processed foods is a great place to start. Look at the labels on notoriously salty foods such as deli meat, condiments, dressings, sauces, canned foods, frozen foods and salty snacks. Choose versions with less salt, or make your own at home!

We've set some sodium thresholds for the recipes our book, never exceeding 800 mg in an entrée or 500 mg in soup. To do that, we cooked exclusively with no-salt-added versions of broth and canned beans, used sodium-reduced tamari (instead of soy sauce) and added tons of herbs and spices for flavour.

When you're tasting a recipe, you may like more (or less) salt than what we've recommended, and that's okay! Taste is subjective, and, as noted previously, taste is paramount. Don't be afraid to add an extra sprinkle of salt. It's not the main culprit that's affecting your daily sodium intake. If you cut back on processed foods and cook from scratch more often, your sodium intake will naturally be reduced.

A Note About Broth

Our recipes are made with no-salt-added vegetable broth so we can control the amount of sodium in the final soups, stews and chilies that we make. We used the Campbell's No Salt Added Vegetable Broth because it has a delicious, mildly sweet flavour and is easy to locate in all stores. Some soup broths can contain over 4,000 milligrams sodium per container. That's a LOT of salt! It's more nutritious to make your own broth (see page 107), or use a no-salt-added variety and season your final soup bowl to taste. You'll never add as much salt with a few dashes from the salt shaker as what you'll find in a full-sodium packaged broth, bouillon cube or soup powder.

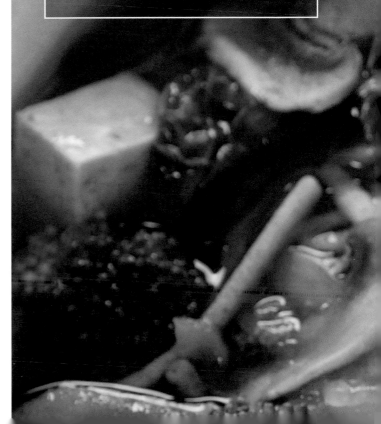

FISH TACOS WITH CORN SALSA, P. 141

CHAPTER

7

Entrées

Tip: An ovenproof skillet is a pan that can go from stovetop right into the oven, and is safe to use at high temperatures. It does not have a plastic handle that will melt or scorch. We used a cast iron skillet and had excellent results.

Sesame-Crusted Salmon with Asian Greens & Tamari Dressing

The sesame seed crust adds terrific crunch to the tender salmon and locks the moisture in. The combination of black and white sesame seeds on the bed of greens adds a visually appealing colour contrast to this delectable meal. It's an impressive plate to prepare for company. —Cara

1. Preheat oven to 400°F (200°C).

2. Add brown rice and water to a medium-sized pot set over high heat. Bring to a boil uncovered. Once boiling, reduce heat to medium-low, cover, and simmer for 45–50 minutes or until tender. Add more water if necessary so rice does not burn. Or, alternately, cook in a rice steamer.

3. Combine the white and black sesame seeds and salt on a plate. Press each salmon fillet in the seeds to evenly coat one side. Heat 1 Tbsp (15 mL) of the oil in a large, ovenproof skillet over medium heat. Cook the salmon, seed side down, for 5 minutes. Transfer to preheated oven and cook for 10 minutes, or until fish is opaque and flakes easily with a fork.

4. Heat the remaining 1 Tbsp (15 mL) oil in a large wok or skillet over medium heat. Add the ginger and garlic and stir-fry for 1 minute. Add the bok choy and stir-fry for 5 minutes or until almost wilted.

5. To make the tamari dressing, in a small bowl, whisk together hoisin, tamari and vinegar. Stir well. Add half the dressing to the bok choy. Toss to combine.

6. To serve, divide the rice among serving plates, top with bok choy and one piece of salmon, and drizzle the remaining dressing on top.

SERVES 4

1 cup (250 mL) long-grain brown rice

1½ cups (500 mL) water

2 Tbsp (30 mL) white sesame seeds

2 Tbsp (30 mL) black sesame seeds

⅛ tsp (0.5 mL) sea salt

4 fillets (6 oz/170 g each) salmon, skinless

2 Tbsp (30 mL) extra virgin olive oil, divided

10 cups (2.5 L) washed and chopped bok choy

One 1-inch (2.5 cm) piece fresh ginger, minced

2 garlic cloves, minced

Tamari dressing

3 Tbsp (45 mL) sodium-reduced hoisin sauce

3 Tbsp (45 mL) sodium-reduced tamari

1½ Tbsp (22 mL) rice vinegar

NUTRIENTS PER SERVING SERVING SIZE: ¼ RECIPE

611 calories, 30 g fat, 5 g saturated fat, 740 mg sodium, 50 g carbohydrates, 7 g fibre, 7 g sugars, 37 g protein. Very high in fibre. Excellent source thiamin, niacin, folate, vitamin B$_6$, vitamin C, vitamin D, vitamin B$_{12}$ and magnesium. Good source of vitamin A, folate, calcium and iron.

Quinoa Chili with Kidney Beans

Dry roasting quinoa brings out the natural nutty flavour of the grain. My husband, Jim, has added squash, chicken, asparagus, flank steak, you name it, to this chili recipe. He thinks the chili powder–tomato sauce combination is a good flavour base for most recipes. He also adds more stock to his bowl when he wants a more "soupy" texture. —Nettie

1. In a skillet over medium heat, roast the rinsed quinoa for 5 minutes or until fragrant and the quinoa begins to pop.

2. In a small pot, bring water to boil. Add roasted quinoa. Cover and simmer over medium heat for 15 minutes. Remove from the heat, let stand covered for 5 minutes then fluff with a fork. Set aside.

3. Heat oil in large pot over medium heat. Cook onion and garlic for 5 minutes or until softened. Stir in mushrooms, green pepper, celery, chili powder, oregano, paprika, salt and pepper. Cook for 8 minutes, stirring often.

4. Stir in tomatoes and beans. Simmer for 10 minutes, stirring occasionally.

5. Stir in the quinoa and green onions. Continue heating on low heat for 5 minutes or until chili is hot.

NUTRIENTS PER SERVING
SERVING SIZE: ⅙ RECIPE

276 calories, 7 g fat, 1 g saturated fat, 744 mg sodium, 46 g carbohydrates, 13 g fibre, 11 g sugars, 11 g protein. Very high in fibre. Excellent source of vitamin A, folate, vitamin C, magnesium and iron.

SERVES 6

1 cup (250 mL) quinoa, rinsed

2 cups (500 mL) water

2 Tbsp (30 mL) extra virgin olive oil

1 onion, diced

3 garlic cloves, minced

1 cup (250 mL) thinly sliced button mushrooms

1 green pepper, seeded and thinly sliced

1 celery stalk, diced

1 Tbsp (15 mL) chili powder

1 Tbsp (15 mL) dried oregano

2 tsp (10 mL) paprika

½ tsp (2 mL) sea salt

½ tsp (2 mL) freshly ground black pepper

2 cans (28 oz/830 mL each) diced tomatoes

14 oz (410 mL) can no-salt-added red kidney beans, rinsed

2 green onions, sliced

Savoury Chickpea Patties with Tzatziki

Ask most four-year-olds to name their favourite food, and you may hear "pizza" or "ice cream." If you ask my son Aubrey, he'll say "chickpeas!" He's not kidding—he really loves the little legumes, and this is one of my go-to dinner recipes to please his often-picky palate. The savoury tzatziki is the perfect accompaniment to these minty, lemony, full-flavoured patties. They are also perfect for the lunch box. —Cara

1. To make the tzatziki, in a small bowl, combine the cucumber, yogurt, garlic, salt and pepper. Cover and refrigerate while preparing the patties.

2. To make the patties, in the bowl of a food processor, combine 2 Tbsp (30 mL) flaxseed, sesame seeds, chickpeas, oats, garlic and mint. Pulse until the mixture is coarsely chopped. Add the lemon juice, cumin, salt and pepper. Pulse the food processor until the mixture is just combined.

3. Using your hands, shape into small patties, using about ¼ cup (60 mL) of the mixture per patty (it will make 16 patties). If the mixture is too thick, add a tablespoon or two of water and stir to combine.

4. Combine the bread crumbs and remaining 1 Tbsp (15 mL) flaxseed on a plate. Dredge patties in the breadcrumb mixture.

5. In a large non-stick skillet, heat the oil over medium heat. Add the patties and cook for 3–5 minutes per side, or until golden.

6. Serve topped with tzatziki.

 Tip: If you don't have a food processor (or don't feel like digging it out and cleaning it afterwards), this recipe will also work using a hand blender (also called an immersion blender).

NUTRIENTS PER SERVING
SERVING SIZE: 4 PATTIES PLUS ¼ OF TZATZIKI

269 calories, 12 g fat, 2 g saturated fat, 562 mg sodium, 30 g carbohydrates, 8 g fibre, 2 g sugars, 10 g protein. Very high in fibre. Good source of magnesium, iron and zinc.

SERVES 4

Tzatziki
½ medium English cucumber, peeled, seeded and grated
¼ cup (60 mL) 2% Greek yogurt
Pinch of garlic powder
⅛ tsp (0.5 mL) sea salt
⅛ tsp (0.5 mL) freshly ground black pepper

Patties
3 Tbsp (45 mL) ground flaxseed, divided
1 Tbsp (15 mL) raw sesame seeds
14 oz (410 mL) can no-salt-added chickpeas
¼ cup (60 mL) large flake rolled oats
2 garlic cloves, minced
½ cup (125 mL) chopped fresh mint
3 Tbsp (45 mL) fresh lemon juice
2 tsp (10 mL) ground cumin
¾ tsp (4 mL) sea salt
⅛ tsp (0.5 mL) freshly ground black pepper
¼ cup (60 mL) whole grain breadcrumbs
2 Tbsp (30 mL) extra virgin olive oil

Tempeh Noodle Bowl with Cashews

Cashew nuts are so delicious! Their rich, buttery flavour lends itself to the recipe below to create a memorable sauce. We use the cashew butter from a Canadian company called Nuts to You, and the only ingredient is cashews—no added sugar, salt or fat. Mango, cashews and coconut are in perfect harmony in this dish. Cooking the noodles and green beans in the coconut milk imparts a subtle coconut flavour, without the high calorie count. —Nettie

1. To make the sauce, in a small bowl, whisk together cashew butter, tamari, mirin, sesame oil and curry powder. Set aside.

2. In a medium-sized frying pan or wok, heat coconut oil over high heat. Stir-fry tempeh for 8–10 minutes or until golden. Transfer tempeh to sauce. Stir to coat. Set aside.

3. In a medium-sized saucepan, combine the coconut milk and water and bring to a boil. Add the noodles and cook according to package directions. Remove the noodles from the liquid, saving the water–coconut milk mixture. Add to tempeh marinade. Toss with tongs.

4. Place coconut milk-water saucepan back on stove and bring to a simmer.

5. Add green beans to the simmering water–coconut milk mixture. Cook them for 3–5 minutes, or until just tender. Drain. You can save the leftover coconut broth for future soup stock.

6. Add green beans to the noodle-tempeh mixture. Toss to mix.

7. Add cucumber, carrot and red beans. Cover and marinate until serving time; the optimal marinating time is 1 hour.

8. Right before serving, stir in the mango, mint, green onions and sesame seeds.

NUTRIENTS PER SERVING
SERVING SIZE: JUST OVER 1 CUP (250 ML) NOODLES

502 calories, 31 g fat, 19 g saturated fat, 361 mg sodium, 46 g carbohydrates, 9 g fibre, 10 g sugars, 19 g protein. Very high in fibre. Excellent source of vitamin A, vitamin C, vitamin K, magnesium, iron, manganese and copper. Good source of riboflavin and folate.

SERVES 6

Sauce
¼ cup (60 mL) cashew butter

2 Tbsp (30 mL) sodium-reduced tamari

1 Tbsp (15 mL) mirin

1 Tbsp (15 mL) toasted sesame oil

2 tsp (10 mL) curry powder

Noodle bowl
2 Tbsp (30 mL) coconut oil

1 package (8 oz/225 g) tempeh

2 cups (500 mL) coconut milk

1½ cups (500 mL) water

4 oz (110 g) brown rice noodles

2 cups (500 mL) green beans, trimmed and halved crosswise

½ English cucumber, diced

1 carrot, grated

14 oz (410 mL) can small no-salt-added red beans, drained and rinsed

1 ripe mango, 1-inch (2.5 cm) dice (fresh or frozen)

3 Tbsp (45 mL) fresh mint leaves, cut into thin strips

2 green onions, sliced into ½-inch (1 cm) green and white pieces

½ Tbsp (30 mL) sesame seeds, toasted (see page 25)

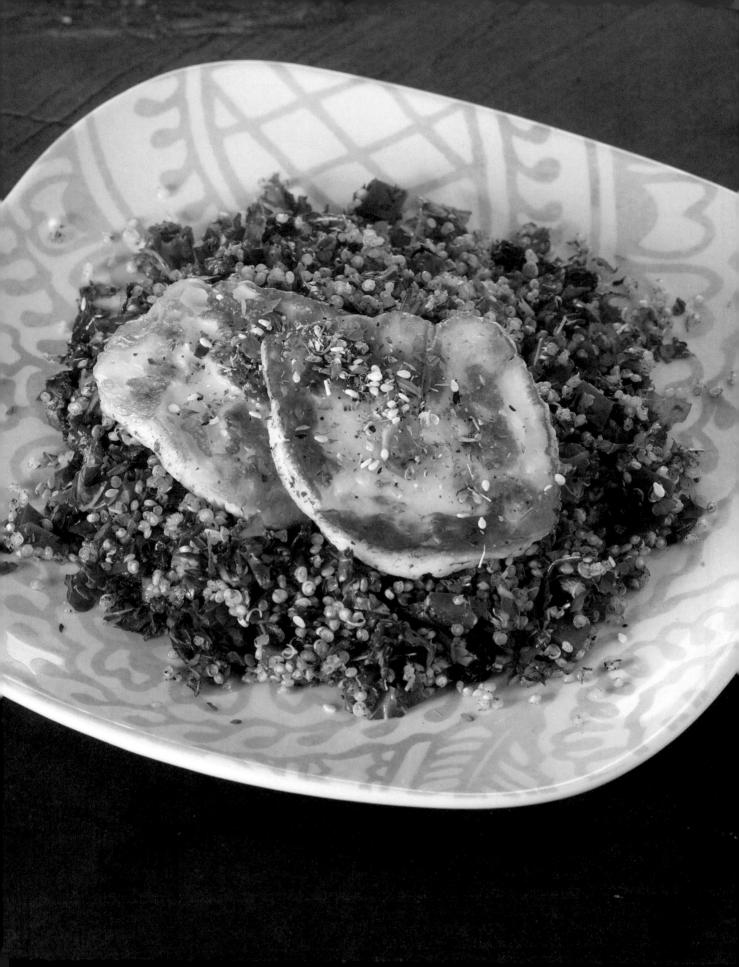

Crisped Halloumi with Za'atar Quinoa

Richly spiced quinoa is the perfect bed for salty halloumi cheese, which is one of the only cheeses you can grill or fry without it melting. The surface of the cheese caramelizes evenly and forms a crisp layer. Kale and red pepper add a pop of colour to this delicious, savoury dish. —Cara

1. To make the quinoa, in a small saucepan, bring quinoa and water to a boil. Reduce heat, cover and simmer 15 minutes. Let sit for 5 minutes, then fluff with a fork.

2. Stir in the lemon zest, cinnamon, za'atar, ¼ cup (60 mL) parsley, sun-dried tomatoes, peppers, kale, olive oil, salt and pepper.

3. To make the crisped halloumi, unwrap the cheese and blot well with paper towel to remove some of the moisture. Cut into eight ¼-inch (6 mm) slices.

4. In a large non-stick pan, heat olive oil over medium heat. Lay slices of cheese in the pan and cook about 5 minutes. Flip and cook on the second side until browned, an additional 3 minutes. The cheese should develop a golden brown colour on each side. Transfer to a plate and sprinkle with lemon juice.

5. To assemble, scoop one cup of quinoa onto a plate. Lay 2 slices of halloumi on top. Serve by finishing with a sprinkling of za'atar and the remaining parsley.

 Tip: Halloumi cheese is a semi-firm white cheese that is native to Cyprus and can be bought at most supermarkets.

NUTRIENTS PER SERVING SERVING SIZE: ¼ RECIPE

418 calories, 25 g fat, 11 g saturated fat, 986 mg sodium, 33 g carbohydrates, 4 g fibre, 2 g sugars, 18 g protein. High in fibre. Excellent source of vitamin A, vitamin C, calcium and iron.

SERVES 4

Quinoa

1 cup (250 mL) quinoa, rinsed

2 cups (500 mL) water or no-salt-added vegetable stock

1 tsp (5 mL) lemon zest

1 tsp (5 mL) ground cinnamon

2 Tbsp (30 mL) za'atar (store-bought or see recipe on p138)

½ cup (125 mL) finely chopped fresh parsley, divided

¼ cup (60 mL) chopped sun-dried tomatoes

¼ cup (60 mL) chopped roasted red pepper (from a jar)

2 cups (500 mL) finely chopped kale

1 Tbsp (15 mL) extra virgin olive oil

¼ tsp (1 mL) sea salt

Pinch of freshly ground black pepper

Crisped Halloumi

½ lb (225 g) halloumi cheese

1 Tbsp (15 mL) extra virgin olive oil

1 Tbsp (15 mL) fresh lemon juice

Quick Homemade Za'atar

Za'atar is a very popular spice blend throughout the Middle East. It is a delicious combination of herbs, seeds and salt, and we've included how to make your own here. The difficult ingredient to find is sumac, the powder from the tart berry of the sumac tree. The berry is purple-red and is dried and ground into a powder. This powder is available in specialty stores and some grocery stores. If you can't find it, add some pepper and lemon zest to the final plate. You can also find pre-mixed za'atar in the spice section, if you prefer not to make your own. —Nettie

1. In a spice grinder or with a mortar and pestle, combine thyme, oregano, sesame, sumac and salt. Pulse or grind until you break up the seeds and have a coarse powder. Store in an airtight container in the fridge and use within 1 week.

2 Tbsp (30 mL) dried thyme

2 Tbsp (30 mL) dried oregano

2 Tbsp (30 mL) sesame seeds, toasted (see page 25)

1 Tbsp (15 mL) ground sumac

¼ tsp (1 mL) kosher salt

A Note About Building a Balanced Meal

A common myth is that it is difficult to eat right because planning well-balanced meals is hard to do. The truth? Many people are not sure where to start—but once you get the hang of it, it's easy!

One sure-fire method to proper meal planning is to follow the "Plate Rule." When you are thinking about a meal, visualize your dinner plate as having four quadrants. Fill two of these quadrants with your favourite vegetables, from stir-fried greens to roasted veggies to salad. Fill one quadrant with protein-rich food, such as chicken, Greek yogurt, legumes or fish. Fill the final quadrant with whole grains like quinoa or brown rice. It's such a simple way to make sure your meal is well-balanced and delicious.

When you are not using a plate (say you are eating a bowl of hearty soup or stew, for example), you can still make sure you include these elements in the same proportions— ½ vegetables, ¼ whole grains and ¼ protein.

Chickpea Ratatouille on Creamy Parmesan Millet

Sunday brunch with my parents has been a family tradition since my daughter was born. When my mom deviated from the bagels and tuna, she'd add my favourite comfort food to the table and surprise me with her famous ratatouille. And she didn't need to tell me—as soon as I walked in, I could smell the rich tomato broth simmering with eggplant, zucchini and fresh herbs. "Ratatouille??" I'd ask, with an excited smile. And I knew she made it with love—I could taste it. I've added chickpeas to her recipe, and serve it on creamy millet to turn what was once a side dish into a whole meal. With love. —Cara

1. To make the millet, in a small saucepan, bring millet and broth to a boil over high heat. Reduce heat to low, cover and simmer, stirring occasionally for 20–25 minutes or until thick and creamy, adding a little water if it looks dry. Add Parmesan, salt and pepper. Stir to combine. Set aside.

2. To make the ratatouille, heat the olive oil in a large pan over medium heat. Add onion and garlic and cook, stirring occasionally, for 5 minutes or until softened.

3. Add red pepper, zucchini, eggplant and chickpeas and cook, stirring occasionally, for 5 minutes or until vegetables are golden. Add tomatoes and thyme, reduce heat and simmer for 20 minutes or until vegetables are tender, adding a little water if the sauce becomes too thick.

4. To serve, divide the millet among 4 shallow bowls, top with ratatouille and sprinkle with coarsely grated Parmesan.

 Tip: If you don't have fresh thyme, you can use fresh parsley or basil. Or, substitute 2 tsp (10 mL) fresh thyme with ½ tsp (2 mL) dried thyme.

NUTRIENTS PER SERVING SERVING SIZE: ¼ RECIPE

536 calories, 18 g fat, 6 g saturated fat, 717 mg sodium, 72 g carbohydrates, 13 g fibre, 12 g sugars, 24 g protein. Very high in fibre. Excellent source of thiamin, riboflavin, vitamin B₆, folate, vitamin B₁₂, vitamin C, calcium, magnesium, iron and zinc. Good source of niacin.

SERVES 4

Millet

1 cup (250 mL) millet

2 cups (500 mL) no-salt-added vegetable broth

⅔ cup (150 mL) finely grated Parmesan cheese

¼ tsp (1 mL) sea salt

⅛ tsp (0.5 mL) freshly ground black pepper

Ratatouille

2 Tbsp (30 mL) extra virgin olive oil

1 red onion, diced

2 garlic cloves, minced

1 red pepper, diced

1 medium zucchini, diced

1 small eggplant, diced

14 oz (410 mL) can no-salt-added chickpeas

14 oz (410 mL) can chopped tomatoes

2 tsp (10 mL) fresh thyme leaves

½ cup (125 mL) coarsely grated Parmesan cheese

Tip: Don't forget to zest the lime before you juice it—it's difficult to zest it after it has been cut and squeezed!

Fish Tacos with Corn Salsa

I love fish tacos and will order them whenever they appear on a menu. I was inspired to make them at home after enjoying a dinner party with my friends Sari and James. They cooked up restaurant-quality fish tacos, including homemade salsa and guacamole! I began experimenting with my own recipe and learned that fish tacos are a quick weeknight meal once you identify the key ingredients. Seasoning the fish with the right spicy-savoury mix is essential, and fresh cilantro is the crowning glory, so have lots of it around. —Cara

1. Preheat grill to high heat.
2. To make salsa, in a medium bowl, mix together corn, tomato, red onion, jicama, cilantro and pumpkin seeds. Stir in lime juice, zest and salt. Set aside.
3. To prepare fish, in a small bowl, combine cayenne pepper, oregano, paprika and salt. Brush each fish fillet with olive oil, and sprinkle with spices.
4. Arrange fillets on grill grate, and cook for about 6 minutes, or until fish flakes easily with a fork.
5. To serve, build the tacos. For each taco, top corn tortillas with fish, salsa, yogurt and extra cilantro.

SERVES 6

Salsa

1 cup (250 mL) corn kernels

1 large tomato, diced

½ red onion, diced

1 jicama, peeled and diced

½ cup (125 mL) chopped fresh cilantro leaves

¼ cup (60 mL) raw unsalted pumpkin seeds

½ tsp (2 mL) lime zest

2 Tbsp (30 mL) fresh lime juice

½ tsp (2 mL) sea salt

Fish

¼ tsp (1 mL) cayenne pepper, or more if you like it very spicy

1½ tsp (2 mL) dried oregano

½ tsp (2 mL) paprika

½ tsp (2 mL) salt

6 fillets (4 oz/110 g each) tilapia, haddock or catfish

1 tsp (5 mL) extra virgin olive oil

12 corn tortillas (4 inches/10 cm)

2 Tbsp (30 mL) 2% Greek yogurt

½ cup (125 mL) fresh cilantro leaves

Tip: Jicama, also known as Mexican potato, is a white-fleshed tuber with tan-brown skin. It's peeled before being eaten, and can be used both raw and cooked. Either way, it retains a phenomenal crunch and a mild sweetness, reminiscent of a mellow apple or pear. If you can't find it, the salsa is equally good without it!

NUTRIENTS PER SERVING SERVING SIZE: 2 TACOS

251 calories, 7 g fat, 2 g saturated fat, 362 mg sodium, 20 g carbohydrates, 4 g fibre, 4 g sugars, 28 g protein. High in fibre. Excellent source of vitamin B_{12}, vitamin D and magnesium. Good source of niacin.

Colourful Vegetable & Bean Linguine

To make this pasta stand out, the smoked paprika is an essential ingredient. It comes in three varieties: sweet, bittersweet and hot. I recommend the sweet if you have the choice. —Nettie

1. Bring a large pot of water to boil, then cook linguine according to package directions. Set aside.

2. Heat the oil in a large sauté pan over medium heat. Add onion, garlic and oregano, and sauté until onion is translucent, about 4 minutes. Add smoked paprika and sauté a few minutes more.

3. Stir in the cauliflower and season with salt. Sauté until lightly browned, about 4 minutes.

4. Add the tomatoes, kidney beans and collard greens. Bring to a simmer, cover and cook until cauliflower is tender and collard greens are wilted, about 5 minutes. Stir in half of the Asiago cheese.

5. Place the linguine back in the pot or a warmed serving bowl and toss in the sauce to coat the pasta. Serve, topped with parsley and remaining Asiago.

Tip: Whole grain noodles can be made from wheat, corn, brown rice, rice, buckwheat, quinoa or a variety of other nutritious grains. New to the market are noodles made exclusively from bean or lentil flours too! You should experiment to find your favourite. Soba noodles and brown rice noodles would also work well in this dish.

SERVES 6

6 oz 1 box (13 oz/375 g) whole grain linguine

1½ 3 Tbsp (45 mL) extra virgin olive oil

¼ ½ red onion, finely diced

1 2 garlic cloves, minced

½ 1 Tbsp (15 mL) fresh oregano leaves

½ 1 Tbsp (15 mL) smoked paprika

1¼ 2½ cups (500 mL) sliced *Broccoli* cauliflower florets (¼ inch/6 mm)

⅛ ¼ tsp (1 mL) sea salt

1½ 3 cups (750 mL) halved grape or cherry tomatoes

7 oz 14 oz (410 mL) can no-salt-added red kidney beans, drained and rinsed

1½ c 3 cups (750 mL) chopped collard greens *Spinach, Kale*

½ 1 cup (250 mL) grated Asiago cheese, divided

⅛ c ¼ cup (60 mL) fresh Italian parsley leaves

NUTRIENTS PER SERVING
SERVING SIZE: 1¾ CUPS (425 ML) PASTA

463 calories, 16 g fat, 5 g saturated fat, 225 mg sodium, 67 g carbohydrates, 15 g fibre, 8 g sugars, 20 g protein. Very high in fibre. Excellent source of vitamin C, folate and magnesium. Good source of calcium and iron.

Zucchini, Tomato & Olive Tart

This wonderful tart has layers of flavour and colour. While the tart shell we use is homemade, you can skip this step for a quicker recipe and use a store-bought shell. Try to find one that's made without shortening or lard, and whole grain if possible! Colby cheese is similar to cheddar, and can be substituted if you prefer it. —Nettie

1. Preheat the oven to 350°F (180°C).
2. To make the dough, combine the flour and ½ tsp (2 mL) salt in a large bowl. Using pastry cutter or metal fork, cut in the cold butter. Add 1 Tbsp (15 mL) of olive oil and continue cutting until the mixture is sandy in consistency. Add water, a little at a time, just enough to hold the dough together. Form the dough into a soft ball, wrap in plastic wrap and refrigerate for 10 minutes or until ready to use (up to 2 days).
3. Transfer dough to a work surface dusted with flour. Roll dough to ¼ inch (3 mm) thickness, then transfer to an 8-inch (20 cm) tart pan and press it gently into the pan, trimming away any excess if necessary.
4. Bake tart shell for 8–10 minutes, until lightly golden. Remove from oven and let cool.
5. To make the filling, in a medium bowl, toss the zucchini and red beans with oil, salt and pepper.
6. Layer the zucchini and bean mixture onto the tart shell. Sprinkle with olives and lay tomato slices on top. Add colby cheese on top. Bake for 30 minutes. Remove from oven and sprinkle with basil.
7. Cut into six slices and serve.

NUTRIENTS PER SERVING SERVING SIZE: ⅙ RECIPE

301 calories, 17 g fat, 7 g saturated fat, 668 mg sodium, 27 g carbohydrates, 9 g fibre, 2 g sugars, 12 g protein. Very high in fibre. Good source of calcium.

SERVES 6

Dough

1 cup (250 mL) whole grain spelt flour, plus more for dusting

½ tsp (2 mL) sea salt

2 Tbsp (30 mL) unsalted butter, cold

1 Tbsp (15 mL) extra virgin olive oil

2–3 Tbsp (45 mL) cold water

Filling

1 green zucchini, cut into ⅛-inch (3 mm) rounds

1 yellow zucchini, cut into ⅛ inch (3 mm) rounds

14 oz (410 mL) can no-salt-added red beans

1 Tbsp (15 mL) extra virgin olive oil

½ tsp (2 mL) sea salt

¼ tsp (1 mL) freshly ground black pepper

⅓ cup (75 mL) sliced green olives with pimentos

1 medium tomato, cut into six ¼-inch (6 mm) slices

1 cup (250 mL) grated colby cheese

¼ cup (60 mL) chopped fresh basil

Grilled Vegetable & Goat Cheese Sandwiches

As my friends know, if a sandwich like this appears on any restaurant menu, I will order it. Crunchy bread, melty goat cheese, tender grilled vegetables and garlicky pesto are such a spectacular combination that I had to create my own version of this dish at home. Adding white beans to the pesto gives it an extra-smooth texture, and the kale . . . well, I add kale wherever I can! Despite the long instruction list, it's incredibly easy to make this at home—and now my friends want to skip the restaurant and come here for lunch. —Cara

1. To prepare the pesto, in a large pan, add 1 Tbsp (15 mL) olive oil and garlic. Once sizzling, add kale and sauté 5 for minutes. Remove from heat.

2. Add kale to food processor bowl, along with remaining oil, walnuts, lemon juice, salt, beans, Parmesan and basil. Pulse all ingredients together until mixture becomes creamy.

3. Adjust salt and lemon juice to taste. Refrigerate until ready to use. Excess can be stored for 3 days.

4. To prepare the grilled vegetables, preheat grill to medium-high heat.

5. Brush eggplant, zucchini and red pepper with olive oil and season with salt and pepper.

6. Grill until just tender—about 8 minutes for the eggplant and zucchini, and 10 minutes for the pepper.

7. To prepare the sandwiches, start by toasting bread.

8. Spread 1 Tbsp (15 mL) of pesto each on of four slices of bread.

9. Lay slices of eggplant, zucchini and red pepper atop the pesto.

10. Divide arugula evenly between sandwiches.

11. Spread 2 Tbsp (30 mL) goat cheese over each of four remaining bread slices; place, cheese side down, on sandwiches.

SERVES 6

Pesto

¼ cup (60 mL) extra virgin olive oil, divided

1 garlic clove, minced

6 cups (1.5 L) chopped Tuscan kale

¼ cup (60 mL) chopped walnuts

2 Tbsp (30 mL) fresh lemon juice

½ tsp (2 mL) sea salt

14 oz (410 mL) can no-salt-added cannellini beans

¼ cup (60 mL) grated Parmesan cheese

¼ cup (60 mL) fresh basil leaves

Grilled vegetables

1 Japanese eggplant, cut into ¼-inch (6mm) thick slices

1 zucchini, cut into ¼-inch (6 mm) thick slices

1 red pepper, cut into 2-inch (5 cm) strips

2 Tbsp (30 mL) extra virgin olive oil

¼ tsp (1 mL) sea salt

⅛ tsp (0.5 mL) freshly ground black pepper

Sandwiches

8 slices whole grain bread or baguette

1 cup (250 mL) baby arugula

4.5 oz (130 g) soft goat cheese

NUTRIENTS PER SERVING SERVING SIZE: 1 SANDWICH

402 calories, 22 g fat, 8 g saturated fat, 711 mg sodium, 40 g carbohydrates, 7 g fibre, 8 g sugars, 16 g protein. Very high in fibre. Excellent source of folate and vitamin C. Good source of vitamin A, riboflavin, calcium, magnesium and iron.

Tip: The leftover pesto makes a perfect sauce for pasta, or can be frozen and used as needed.

Fajita Quesadillas

This recipe is a crowd pleaser. When my son Emery's hockey teammates drop in for a pre-game dinner, we serve this. The boys tailor-make fajitas to suit their taste buds. In addition to beans and cheese, you can also add chicken and steak. —Nettie

1. Heat 1 Tbsp (15 mL) olive oil in a large non-stick skillet pan over medium heat. Add peppers, onion and mushroom and cook for 10 minutes or until softened. Add beans and warm through, about 2 minutes.
2. On one tortilla, arrange one-quarter each of the cooked vegetables and beans, cheese and green onions. Top with a second tortilla.
3. Heat remaining oil in skillet over medium heat. Cook the quesadilla 2–4 minutes on each side or until tortillas are golden brown and cheese has melted.
4. Cut each quesadilla into quarters and top with avocado, salsa and Greek yogurt.

Tip: You can freeze any leftover quesadillas individually. Cut pieces of parchment paper to suit the size of the quesadillas and place a piece of paper in between them, then add to a freezer-safe resealable bag or container.

MAKES 12 QUESADILLAS

2 Tbsp (30 mL) extra virgin olive oil, divided

1 yellow pepper, seeded and julienned

1 red pepper, julienned

½ red onion, julienned

1 cup (250 mL) sliced button mushrooms

14 oz (410 mL) can no-salt-added small red beans, drained

12 whole grain flour tortillas (6 inches/15 cm)

1 cup (250 mL) cheddar cheese, grated

4 green onions, cut on the bias (green parts only)

2 ripe avocados, sliced

½ cup (125 mL) salsa

¼ cup (60 mL) 2% Greek yogurt

NUTRIENTS PER SERVING
SERVING SIZE: 2 QUESADILLAS

480 calories, 25 g fat, 6 g saturated fat, 658 mg sodium, 49 g carbohydrates, 14 g fibre, 3 g sugars, 18 g protein. Very high in fibre. Excellent source of folate and vitamin C. Good source of riboflavin, vitamin B_6, calcium, magnesium, iron and zinc.

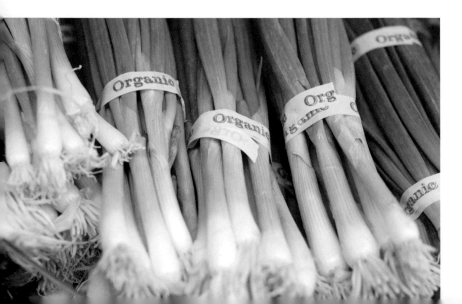

Refried Bean Tacos with Broccoli Slaw

This recipe is quick and convenient for busy weeknights, since it relies on healthy packaged (not processed!) foods that are simple to assemble. When buying canned refried beans, read the label. Be aware of salt content and added fat (such as lard), especially if you want your beans for a vegetarian meal. We used Eden Refried Beans because they are low in sodium and are made without lard. Pre-shredded broccoli or cabbage slaw (with no added salad dressing) can be found in the bagged salad aisle in every grocery store. —Nettie

1. In a medium-sized bowl, combine the slaw, carrots and cilantro. Add 2 Tbsp (30 mL) olive oil, lime juice and ⅛ tsp (1 mL) salt to slaw. Toss well. Set aside.

2. In a small bowl, combine refried beans, salsa, green onion, chili powder, cumin and remaining salt.

3. Divide the refried bean mixture among the tortillas, filling about one-third full. Fold tortillas in half and press down gently.

4. Heat 1 Tbsp (15 mL) of olive oil in a large non-stick skillet over medium heat. Add 2 tortillas to the pan and cook until golden brown on each side, about 2 minutes per side. Remove tortilla from heat. Repeat for the remaining tortillas.

5. Gently peel back the warm tortilla and stuff each one with slaw and feta cheese.

6. Serve warm.

Tip: Broccoli slaw is a great time saver. Most people toss broccoli stems, but once the outer layer of tough skin is peeled away, the inner core is a tender vegetable that can be shredded like cabbage to make a lovely slaw. Buying it pre-shredded is a great time saver.

SERVES 4

2 cups (500 mL) broccoli slaw or cabbage slaw

1 medium carrot, grated

⅓ cup (75 mL) chopped fresh cilantro

¼ cup (60 mL) plus 1 Tbsp (15 mL) extra virgin olive oil, divided

1 Tbsp (15 mL) fresh lime juice

¼ tsp (1 mL) sea salt, divided

14 oz (410 mL) can no-salt-added refried beans

½ cup (125 mL) salsa

1 green onion, chopped

1 tsp (5 mL) chili powder

1 tsp (5 mL) ground cumin

8 corn tortillas (4 inches/10 cm each)

½ cup (125 mL) crumbled feta cheese, crumbled

NUTRIENTS PER SERVING SERVING SIZE: 2 TACOS

366 calories, 20 g fat, 4 g saturated fat, 552 mg sodium, 36 g carbohydrates, 12 g fibre, 4 g sugars, 12 g protein. Very high in fibre. Good source of vitamin A.

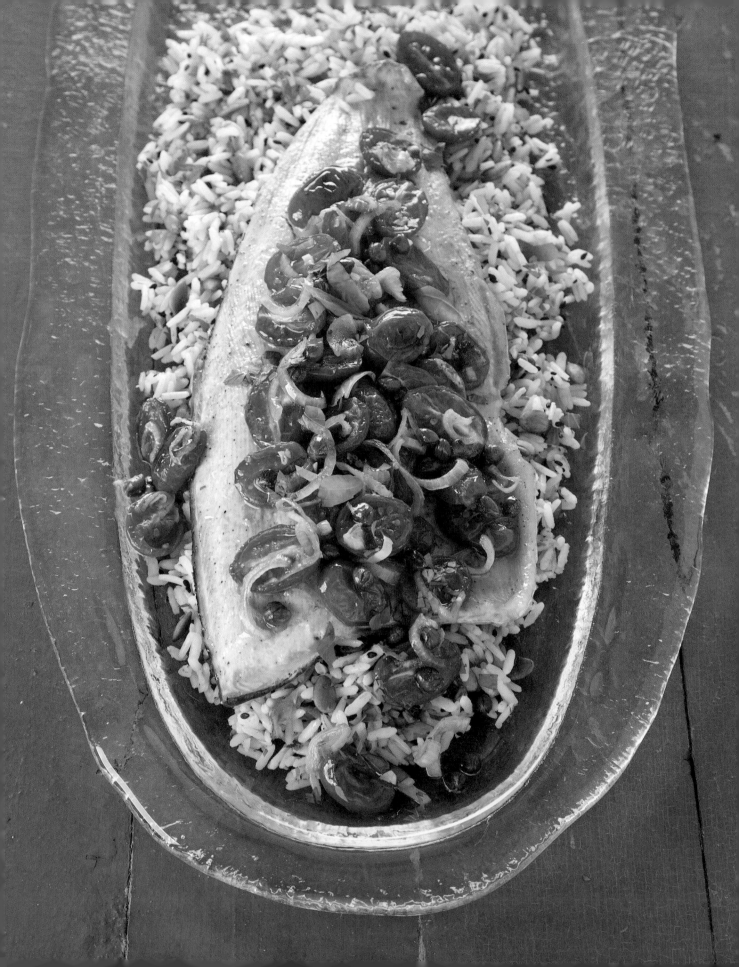

Baked Trout & Tomatoes

When you hear about heart-healthy omega-3 fats, you may automatically think of salmon, but rainbow trout can also be your go-to fish, since it has almost as much omega-3 fat. The sweet roasted tomatoes and salty capers are the perfect accompaniment to this delicate fish. —Cara

1. Preheat the oven to 400°F (200°C). Line a rimmed baking sheet with parchment paper.

2. In a small bowl, toss the tomatoes with shallot, capers, vinegar, oil and ¼ tsp (1 mL) salt. Pour onto baking sheet and bake for 30 minutes.

3. Cook brown rice according to package directions, about 10–15 minutes.

4. Season the trout with the remaining salt, pepper and mustard. After the tomatoes have roasted for 30 minutes, remove the baking sheet from the oven and add the trout. Continue to bake for 10 more minutes, or until fish flakes easily with a fork.

5. Add sesame seeds, pumpkin seeds, salt, basil and parsley to rice. Toss to combine.

6. Sprinkle remaining parsley and basil over trout. Serve trout over rice.

A Note About Brown Rice

Brown rice is a whole grain. The rice kernel has not been stripped of its brown seed coat, which means that the nutritious grain still contains the fibre-rich bran, vitamin-heavy germ and starchy endosperm. White rice is devoid of those healthy layers, and just the endosperm is left. The downside of all that whole grain goodness? It takes about 50 minutes to cook! But there is an option for making brown rice in a fraction of that time, which we use here: parboiled rice. We tried Uncle Ben's, which cooks in 10–15 minutes. It worked so well!

SERVES 6

2 cups (500 mL) halved grape tomatoes

1 medium shallot, thinly sliced

1 Tbsp (15 mL) capers, drained

2 Tbsp (30 mL) red wine vinegar

2 Tbsp (30 mL) extra virgin olive oil

½ tsp (2 mL) sea salt, divided

6 fillets (4 oz/110 g each) rainbow trout fillets

⅛ tsp (0.5 mL) freshly ground pepper

2 Tbsp (30 mL) Dijon mustard

1 Tbsp (15 mL) chopped fresh parsley

1 Tbsp (15 mL) chopped fresh basil

Brown Rice

1 cup (250 mL) parboiled brown rice (see tip, left)

2 Tbsp (30 mL) black sesame seeds

2 Tbsp (30 mL) raw unsalted pumpkin seeds

¼ tsp (1 mL) sea salt

1 Tbsp (15 mL) chopped fresh basil

1 Tbsp (15 mL) chopped fresh flat-leaf parsley

NUTRIENTS PER SERVING SERVING SIZE: ⅙ RECIPE

251 calories, 7 g fat, 2 g saturated fat, 362 mg sodium, 20 g carbohydrates, 4 g fibre, 4 g sugars, 28 g protein. High in fibre. Excellent source of vitamin B$_{12}$, vitamin D and magnesium. Good source of niacin.

Eggplant Parmesan Pizza

I love eggplant on pizza, or anywhere else for that matter. For a deep-dish-style crust on this pizza, we used extra thick flax pitas. If you prefer thin crust, you can also make this recipe using thin pitas or tortillas. And if you don't feel like ricotta cheese, goat cheese works equally well. —Cara

1. Preheat oven to 450°F (220°C).
2. Arrange eggplant in a single layer on a foil-lined, greased baking sheet; bake for about 15 minutes turning once, until golden.
3. Spread tomato sauce on pitas and sprinkle with mozzarella cheese.
4. Dollop each pita with ricotta cheese, followed by tomatoes and eggplant. Sprinkle with Parmesan and pine nuts.
5. Bake for about 10 minutes or until golden brown. Sprinkle with fresh basil.

 Tip: Instead of baking the eggplant, you can make it on an indoor grill pan or on the barbecue.

SERVES 4

1 large eggplant, sliced in ¼-inch (6 mm) rounds

¾ cup (175 mL) tomato sauce

4 whole grain flax pitas

¾ cup (175 mL) shredded part-skim mozzarella cheese

½ cup (125 mL) part-skim ricotta cheese

2 large tomatoes, sliced

1 Tbsp (15 mL) grated Parmesan cheese

3 Tbsp (45 mL) pine nuts

2 Tbsp (30 mL) shredded basil leaves

NUTRIENTS PER SERVING SERVING SIZE: 1 PITA PIZZA

523 calories, 17 g fat, 5 g saturated fat, 0 g trans fat, 25 mg cholesterol, 790 mg sodium, 72 g carbohydrates, 11 g fibre, 12 g sugars, 23 g protein. Very high in fibre. Excellent source calcium and iron. Good source of folate, vitamin B$_{12}$ and zinc.

Flank Steak with Chimichurri

One of the goals of this book is to show you how beans, nuts and seeds can be used as a satisfying main dish, or in this case, as a complementary accent to an entrée. The chimichurri has a luxurious thickness thanks to the pumpkin seeds, and most people don't think of pairing seeds with steak. We did, and the result is wonderful. —Cara

SERVES 6

Chimichurri marinade

⅓ cup (75 mL) red wine vinegar

3 garlic cloves, minced

1 cup (250 mL) chopped fresh cilantro

1½ cup (125 mL) chopped fresh flat-leaf parsley

2 Tbsp (30 mL) raw unsalted pumpkin seeds

⅔ cup (150 mL) extra virgin olive oil

¼ tsp (1 mL) cayenne

¼ tsp (1 mL) ground cumin

½ tsp (2 mL) sea salt

Flank steak

1½ lb (700 g) flank steak

¼ tsp (1 mL) freshly ground black pepper

Kosher or coarse salt, to taste

1. To prepare the chimichurri marinade, into the bowl of a food processor add vinegar, garlic, cilantro, parsley, pumpkin seeds, oil, cayenne, cumin and salt. Pulse until herbs are finely chopped.

2. Remove ½ cup (125 mL) chimichurri marinade to a small bowl and reserve as sauce.

3. Score both sides of the steak with a sharp knife, making ¼-inch (6 mm) deep knife cuts an inch (2.5 cm) apart. Add steak and remaining marinade to a large freezer bag, seal bag, and turn to coat the steak well. Chill and marinate for at least 1 hour or overnight.

4. Preheat grill to medium-high.

5. Remove steak from marinade and sprinkle with salt and pepper. This will give you a nice crust.

6. Grill for 5 minutes on each side for medium-rare steak. Adjust cooking times to your preferred level of doneness. It's lean, so grill just a few minutes per side.

7. Remove from the grill and place on a cutting board. Cover with aluminum foil and let rest for 10 minutes.

8. Holding a knife at a 45° angle, thinly slice steak against the grain. Serve topped with the reserved chimichurri sauce.

NUTRIENTS PER SERVING SERVING SIZE: ⅙ RECIPE

363 calories, 28 g fat, 6 g saturated fat, 216 mg sodium, 2 g carbohydrates, 1 g fibre, 0 g sugars, 27 g protein. Excellent source of niacin, vitamin B_6, vitamin B_{12} and zinc. Good source of magnesium and iron.

Moroccan Chicken & Pistachio-Studded Quinoa

In my household, I am the only vegetarian. To save time, I require recipes that are flexitarian, which means that I can make them both with meat and without. I can add my vegetarian protein (tofu) to half of the sauce in my own meat-free skillet. Now that my kids Cameron and Mackenzie are in their twenties, they are eating more vegetarian food than before, and it is their choice rather than my suggestion. On the other hand, my 15-year-old son, Emery, is a committed chicken eater, so for this meal, it's one recipe in two skillets. —Nettie

A Note About Chicken

Boneless skinless chicken takes just minutes to cook in comparison to bone-in chicken pieces. The bone acts as insulation, increasing the cooking time. Boneless chicken breasts and thighs are quick cooking and perfect for getting dinner on the table in a flash.

1. Combine cinnamon, ginger, turmeric and coriander in a small bowl and set aside.

2. In a large non-stick skillet over medium heat, warm the olive oil. Brown chicken for about 5 minutes.

3. Turn chicken and add spice mixture, onion, water, garlic, orange juice and salt. Bring to a boil; cover, reduce heat and simmer for 20–25 minutes, until chicken is no longer pink or reaches an internal temperature of 165°F (74°C).

4. Transfer chicken to plate. Bring liquid in skillet to boil. Boil, stirring occasionally, until most of the liquid is evaporated, about 10 minutes, to create the sauce.

SERVES 6

Chicken

½ tsp (2 mL) ground cinnamon

¼ tsp (1 mL) ground ginger

¼ tsp (1 mL) turmeric

¼ tsp (1 mL) ground coriander

2 Tbsp (30 mL) extra virgin olive oil

4 boneless, skinless chicken breasts (6 oz/170 g each)

1 onion, diced

1 cup (250 mL) water

2 garlic cloves, minced

3 Tbsp (45 mL) fresh orange juice

¼ tsp (1 mL) sea salt

2 Tbsp (30 mL) chopped fresh parsley leaves

Quinoa

1½ cups (500 mL) water

¾ cup (175 mL) quinoa, rinsed

1 Tbsp (15 mL) unsalted butter

2 tsp (10 mL) honey

½ tsp (2 mL) sea salt

½ tsp (2 mL) ground cinnamon

¼ cup (60 mL) shelled pistachios, chopped

⅓ cup (75 mL) chopped dried apricots

⅓ cup (75 mL) chopped fresh mint

¼ cup (60 mL) raw unsalted pumpkin seeds

Asiago cheese, divided

¼ cup (60 mL) fresh flat-leaf parsley leaves

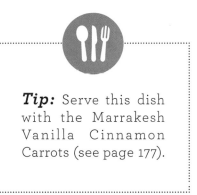

Tip: Serve this dish with the Marrakesh Vanilla Cinnamon Carrots (see page 177).

5. To make the quinoa, in a medium-sized pot, bring water and quinoa to a boil. Reduce heat, cover and simmer for 15 minutes. Remove from heat and set aside for 5 minutes. Fluff with a fork. Toss quinoa with butter, honey, salt, cinnamon, pistachios, apricots, mint and pumpkin seeds.

6. To serve, divide the quinoa among four plates and top each with a piece of chicken. Pour the sauce overtop. Sprinkle with parsley

NUTRIENTS PER SERVING SERVING SIZE: ⅙ RECIPE

404 calories, 17 g fat, 4 g saturated fat, 385 mg sodium, 26 g carbohydrates, 4 g fibre, 8 g sugars, 38 g protein. High in fibre. Excellent source of niacin, vitamin B$_6$, folate, magnesium and zinc. Good source of thiamin and iron.

A Note About Fat

In the mid-1990s, the fat-free craze ruled the fridge and pantry. Hopefully you threw that dietary advice out along with the grunge-inspired flannel shirt and Doc Martens. Fat is good, and fat is essential. You just want to ensure that you choose the right kind of fat for your best health, and don't eat too much of it because the calories add up quickly.

For cooking and salads, I choose extra virgin olive oil most often. It's high in monounsaturated fats, and not too high in any of the more questionable fats. I also have organic canola oil in my pantry, as well as toasted sesame oil for its unique flavour. Butter is used as needed in small amounts—for toast or scrambled eggs or baking cookies, for example. There is no substitute.

Fat from whole foods is also important, and that's why we use nuts and seeds in this book. They are high in good-for-you, heart-healthy fats. Fatty fish, such as

salmon, tuna and trout, contain omega-3 fat, and you should try to eat two servings of these fatty fish each week as well.

Steer clear of foods that contain trans fats, which have the audacity to not only lower our good cholesterol levels, but they raise our bad cholesterol levels too. If you see "partially hydrogenated oil" or "shortening" on an ingredient list, don't buy it. Be especially wary of baked goods like cake, cookies and assorted pastries; that's often where trans fat needlessly lurks. In our book, we use fat from butter, oil, nuts and seeds, and all of the recipes are free of artificial trans fats.

You definitely want to add some type of fat to your salads and vegetables—whether it's oil, nuts, seeds or avocado. Vegetables are rich in antioxidants and phytochemicals, but our bodies require fat to properly absorb them.

Maple-Glazed Lamb Chops with Brussels Sprout–Apple Slaw

The sweet maple syrup glaze and tanginess of the Brussels sprout slaw complements the richness of the lamb. For best results, cook the chops until they are still pink and juicy inside.
—Nettie

1. Cut Brussels sprouts in half lengthwise and then thinly slice each one crosswise.

2. In large bowl, whisk together 1 Tbsp (15 mL) oil, 1 Tbsp (15 mL) vinegar, ¼ tsp (1 mL) salt, and ¼ tsp (1 mL) pepper. Add Brussels sprouts, raisins, seeds and apple. Toss to combine. Set aside.

3. Heat a large skillet over medium-high heat. Sprinkle lamb with remaining salt and pepper. Add remaining oil to pan; swirl to coat. Add lamb to pan; cook for 3 minutes on each side or until done. Remove from pan; keep covered.

4. Add remaining vinegar and maple syrup to pan; bring to a boil. Cook until reduced to 3 Tbsp (45 mL), about 2 minutes. Return lamb to pan. Turn to coat with glaze. Serve with slaw.

Tip: Lamb cuts like chops, racks, loins and tenderloin are quick-to-cook, and taste best when medium-rare. Larger cuts of lamb, such as legs, are best when roasted for longer periods of time.

SERVES 4

12 Brussels sprouts

2 Tbsp (30 mL) extra virgin olive oil, divided

3 Tbsp (45 mL) red wine vinegar, divided

½ tsp (2 mL) sea salt, divided

½ tsp (2 mL) freshly ground black pepper, divided

¼ cup (60 mL) raisins

¼ cup (60 mL) unsalted sunflower seeds, toasted (see page 25)

1 medium Fuji or Gala apple, cut into ⅛-inch (3 mm) thick slices

8 lamb chops (2 oz/60 g each)

2 Tbsp (30 mL) pure maple syrup

NUTRIENTS PER SERVING SERVING SIZE: 2 CHOPS WITH 1½ CUPS (375 ML) SLAW

404 calories, 22 g fat, 8 g saturated fat, 244 mg sodium, 28 g carbohydrates, 4 g fibre, 19 g sugars, 25 g protein. High in fibre. Excellent source of riboflavin, niacin, vitamin B$_{12}$, vitamin C and zinc. Good source of vitamin B$_6$, folate, magnesium and iron.

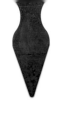

Crispy Kale-Topped Pasta & Cheese Bake

My kids love mac and cheese, and they love kale chips, so I thought I'd try to combine the two! This experiment was a huge success, and my daughter loves to take this to school in her thermos. Make sure to finely chop the kale so it crisps up when baked. For breadcrumbs, I use the thick and crunchy Organic Spelt Breadcrumbs by ShaSha Co. —Cara

1. Preheat oven to 350°F (180°C).
2. Cook pasta according to package directions. Drain pasta and set aside in a large bowl.
3. In a large saucepan over medium heat, melt butter. Add flour, salt and pepper; whisk until well-blended.
4. Pour milk in gradually, while stirring. Bring to a boil for 2 minutes, stirring constantly. Reduce heat and cook for 5 minutes continuing to stir.
5. Over low heat, slowly add 1½ cups cheese, stirring constantly, until it melts. Add nutmeg.
6. Add cheese sauce to pasta, stirring to coat. Transfer to a 9 x 13-inch (23 x 33 cm) baking dish.
7. In a medium bowl, combine the remaining cheese, breadcrumbs, hemp seeds and kale. Stir to combine. Cover the pasta and cheese with the breadcrumb-kale mixture.
8. Bake for 15 minutes until the top is golden brown. You may want to broil for the last 3–4 minutes to get a crispy top. Allow to rest 5 minutes before serving.

SERVES 6

13 oz (375 g) package whole grain penne

2 Tbsp (30 mL) unsalted butter

2 Tbsp (30 mL) whole wheat flour

½ tsp (2 mL) sea salt

⅛ tsp (0.5 mL) freshly ground black pepper

2 cups (500 mL) 2% milk

2 cups (500 mL) shredded cheddar cheese, divided

¼ tsp (1 mL) nutmeg

½ cup (125 mL) whole grain breadcrumbs

¼ cup (60 mL) hemp seeds

2 cups (500 mL) very finely chopped kale

Tip: Adding seeds to the breadcrumbs creates a wonderful crunchy topping. We used hemp seeds, but I've also had great results using chia, ground flax and sesame seeds in this baked dish.

NUTRIENTS PER SERVING SERVING SIZE: ⅙ RECIPE

566 calories, 22 g fat, 12 g saturated fat, 523 mg sodium, 65 g carbohydrates, 8 g fibre, 8 g sugars, 27 g protein. Very high in fibre. Excellent source of vitamin A, thiamin, riboflavin, folate, vitamin B$_{12}$, calcium, magnesium, iron and zinc. Good source of niacin, vitamin C and vitamin D.

Quinoa Tuna Casserole

If you grew up in the 1970s, you've likely eaten your fair share of tuna casserole, probably while wearing bell-bottomed corduroy pants and watching *Charlie's Angels*. Pasta, tuna and a can of Andy Warhol's favourite mushroom soup was comfort food at its best. We've updated that classic staple with modern ingredients that probably weren't in your pantry in 1975: quinoa and flax. Enjoy! —Cara

1. Preheat oven to 375°F (190°C).

2. In a medium saucepan, bring water and quinoa to a boil. Cover, reduce to a simmer and cook for 15 minutes. Remove from heat and fluff with a fork.

3. In a large saucepan, add 1 Tbsp (15 mL) olive oil. Sauté the onion, celery, carrot, red pepper, mushrooms and garlic until tender, about 12–14 minutes. Remove from heat, add quinoa to the vegetable mixture and set aside.

4. To make the sauce, in a medium-sized saucepan over medium heat, combine the remaining 1 Tbsp (15 mL) oil, milk, flour, salt and pepper. Stir until thickened, about 5 minutes. Remove from heat.

5. Add the sauce, tuna, peas and 1 cup (250 mL) of the cheese to the quinoa mixture in the large saucepan. Stir to combine and pour the mixture into a greased 9 x 13–inch (23 x 33 cm) casserole dish. Top with the remaining ½ cup (125 mL) cheese and flaxseeds.

6. Bake for 25 minutes, until bubbling hot. Let cool slightly and serve.

SERVES 6

2 cups (500 mL) water

1 cup (250 mL) quinoa, rinsed

2 Tbsp (30 mL) extra virgin olive oil, divided

¼ onion, diced

1 stalk celery, diced

1 carrot, diced

1 red pepper, diced

2 cups (500 mL) diced button mushrooms

1 garlic clove, minced

2 cups (500 mL) 2% milk

¼ cup (60 mL) whole grain wheat or quinoa flour

½ tsp (2 mL) sea salt

¼ tsp (1 mL) freshly ground black pepper

2 cans (6 oz/170 g each) flaked light tuna, drained (skipjack or yellowfin)

1 cup (250 mL) frozen peas, thawed

1½ cups (375 mL) shredded cheddar cheese

1 Tbsp (15 mL) flaxseeds, ground

A Note About Tuna

Many people prefer the higher-priced white (albacore) tuna when buying canned fish, but this recipe specifically calls for flaked light skipjack or yellowfin tuna. That's because light tuna is lower in mercury than white tuna, and since this is a recipe often served to children, you're better off with a low-mercury fish.

NUTRIENTS PER SERVING SERVING SIZE: JUST OVER 1 CUP (250 ML) CASSEROLE

404 calories, 17 g fat, 4 g saturated fat, 385 mg sodium, 26 g carbohydrates, 4 g fibre, 8 g sugars, 38 g protein.
High in fibre. Excellent source of niacin, vitamin B$_6$, folate, magnesium and zinc. Good source of thiamin and iron.

Chana Masala

This dish appears in the book as a special request from my husband, Scott. A long-time lover of Indian food, he has been a fan of this dish for many years and hoped we'd create a signature version to suit his taste buds (read: extra spicy!) This got an A+ rating—but we doubled the cayenne in his bowl! —Cara

1. In a large frying pan, heat oil over medium heat. Add onion, frying until the edges begin to brown, about 5 minutes.
2. Add the ginger, cumin, coriander, cayenne and turmeric. Stir to combine.
3. Stir in tomatoes and salt.
4. Add water, bring to a boil and simmer, covered, about 10 minutes.
5. Add chickpeas and an additional ½ cup (125 mL) of water. Bring to a boil. Cover, turn heat to low, and simmer for 15 minutes or until water is mostly absorbed. Add a few tablespoons of water if pan is dry.
6. Add garam masala and lemon juice; stir to combine.
7. Add to serving bowls and top with cilantro.

Serve Chana Masala over quinoa, brown basmati rice or millet.

 Tip: If you have leftover chana masala, toss it in the blender with a tablespoon of water or lemon juice for an out-of-this-world variation on hummus.

SERVES 4

3 Tbsp (45 mL) extra virgin olive oil

1 onion, diced

1 tsp (5 mL) grated fresh ginger

1½ tsp (2 mL) ground cumin

1 tsp (5 mL) ground coriander

¼ tsp (1 mL) cayenne (or ½ tsp/2 mL if you like it very spicy)

¼ tsp (1 mL) turmeric

3 plum tomatoes, diced

1 tsp (5 mL) sea salt

1½ cups (500 mL) water, divided

19 oz (560 mL) can no-salt-added chickpeas

½ tsp (2 mL) garam masala

1 tsp (5 mL) fresh lemon juice

¼ cup (60 mL) fresh cilantro leaves, for garnish

NUTRIENTS PER SERVING
SERVING SIZE: ½ CUP (125 ML) CHANA MASALA ONLY

203 calories, 10 g fat, 1 g saturated fat, 456 mg sodium, 24 g carbohydrates, 5 g fibre, 3 g sugars, 7 g protein. High in fibre. Excellent source of folate.

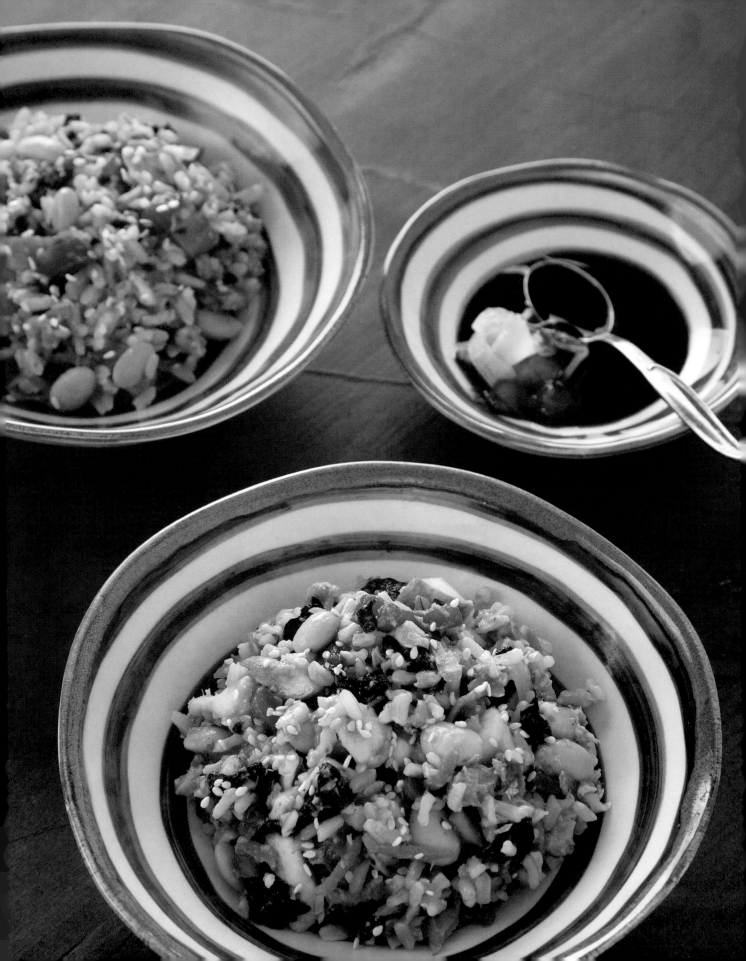

One-Bowl Sushi

These fun and festive rice bowls are like sushi, without the rolling! In this recipe we use brown rice and marinate it with mirin, ginger, tamari and wasabi. Salmon and edamame are protein options; pick your favourite or use them both. Nori is the name for the square-shaped sheets of seaweed used to wrap sushi; in this case, it's torn into bite-sized pieces and stirred into each bowl. —Nettie

1. Rinse brown rice in a fine-mesh colander under cool water, drain. Bring water to a boil in a medium-sized pot over high heat. Stir in rinsed rice. Cover, reduce heat and simmer for 45–50 minutes or until rice is tender. Alternatively, you can use a rice cooker or steamer. Transfer cooked rice to a large bowl.

2. In a small bowl combine vinegar, mirin, ginger, wasabi and tamari. Whisk well to combine. Pour over cooked rice and toss to coat.

3. Add carrot, cucumber, red pepper, avocado, nori, edamame and salmon. Stir to combine.

4. Sprinkle with sesame seeds and serve in bowls.

Tip: You can buy pickled ginger in the condiment or sushi section of the grocery store. Our favourite is the true-to-the-original-colour beige ginger, which is made simply with ginger, salt, vinegar and organic sugar cane. Unlike the bright pink variety of pickled ginger, this one has no trace of artificial sweeteners, food colouring or dye. Once opened it can keep in the refrigerator for up to 2 months.

SERVES 6

1¼ cup (60 mL) short-grain brown rice

2½ cups (625 mL) water

¼ cup (60 mL) rice vinegar

2 Tbsp (30 mL) mirin (Japanese rice wine)

¼ cup (60 mL) pickled ginger, minced

1 tsp (5 mL) wasabi powder

2 Tbsp (30 mL) sodium-reduced tamari

1 carrot, grated

½ English cucumber, diced

1 red pepper, diced

1 ripe avocado, diced

5 sheets nori, torn into bite-sized pieces

1 cup (250 mL) edamame, shelled and boiled according to package directions

1 can (170 g) boneless, skinless salmon

2 Tbsp (30 mL) sesame seeds, toasted (see page 25)

NUTRIENTS PER SERVING
SERVING SIZE: JUST OVER 1 CUP (250 ML) BOWL

308 calories, 9 g fat, 1 g saturated fat, 444 mg sodium, 47 g carbohydrates, 7 g fibre, 5 g sugars, 12 g protein. Very high in fibre. Excellent source of folate and vitamin C. Good source of magnesium.

Seed-Crusted Halibut with Salsa Fresca Penne

The crumbly, crunchy crust on this halibut helps lock in moisture, which results in a juicy and tender fillet. The pasta is ideal with this fresh spring salsa, which can be served hot or cold. It makes a great pasta salad for tomorrow's lunch. —Cara

1. To make the fish, preheat the oven to 400°F (200°C). Line a baking sheet with foil.

2. Combine bread crumbs, hemp seeds, parsley, cilantro, oil, zest, salt and pepper in a bowl. Place halibut fillets onto the prepared baking sheet.

3. Generously spoon the herbed crumbs over the fish, and lightly press crumb mixture onto each fillet with your hands. Bake until crumb topping is lightly browned and fish flakes easily with a fork, about 10–15 minutes.

4. To make the salsa, in a medium bowl, stir together tomatoes, olives, onion, jalapeno, cilantro, parsley, lemon zest and salt. Add olive oil and stir to combine. Set aside.

5. To make the pasta, add penne to a pot of rapidly boiling water. Cook until al dente, about 10–12 minutes. Drain.

6. Place penne in a large bowl. Add salsa to penne and stir.

7. To plate, place pasta with salsa on the plate. Top with crusted halibut.

Tip: The level of heat from the jalapeno depends on how it's cut. Many people think the heat is in the seeds, but that's not quite right. It's actually the ribs that house the seeds, so if you remove the ribs, you will get a slightly milder flavour.

NUTRIENTS PER SERVING SERVING SIZE: ¼ RECIPE

604 calories, 24 g fat, 3 g saturated fat, 777 mg sodium, 52 g carbohydrates, 8 g fibre, 5 g sugars, 44 g protein. Very high in fibre. Excellent source of thiamin, niacin, vitamin B$_6$, folate, vitamin B$_{12}$, magnesium, and iron. Good source of riboflavin, vitamin C and zinc.

SERVES 4

Halibut

½ cup (125 mL) panko bread crumbs

¼ cup (60 mL) hemp seeds

⅓ cup (75 mL) chopped fresh flat-leaf parsley

¼ cup (60 mL) chopped fresh cilantro

2 Tbsp (30 mL) extra virgin olive oil

1 tsp (5 mL) lemon zest

½ tsp (2 mL) sea salt

¼ tsp (1 mL) freshly ground black pepper

4 fillets (6 oz/170 g each) halibut

Salsa fresca

2 medium tomatoes, diced

¼ cup (60 mL) chopped pitted olives

¼ red onion, diced

1 small jalapeno pepper, minced (optional)

½ cup (125 mL) chopped fresh cilantro

2 Tbsp (30 mL) chopped fresh parsley

1 tsp (5 mL) lemon zest

½ tsp (2 mL) sea salt

2 Tbsp (30 mL) extra virgin olive oil

Pasta

2 cups (500 mL) whole grain penne

Tip: When cooked properly, fish is moist and delicate, but many people are afraid of cooking fish at home! The number one preparation error? Overcooking it. Remember this rule: whether you grill, broil, poach, steam, plank or bake fish, cook it 10 minutes per inch, turning it at the halfway point. The halibut we cooked was about 1½ inches (4 cm), and it baked perfectly in 15 minutes.

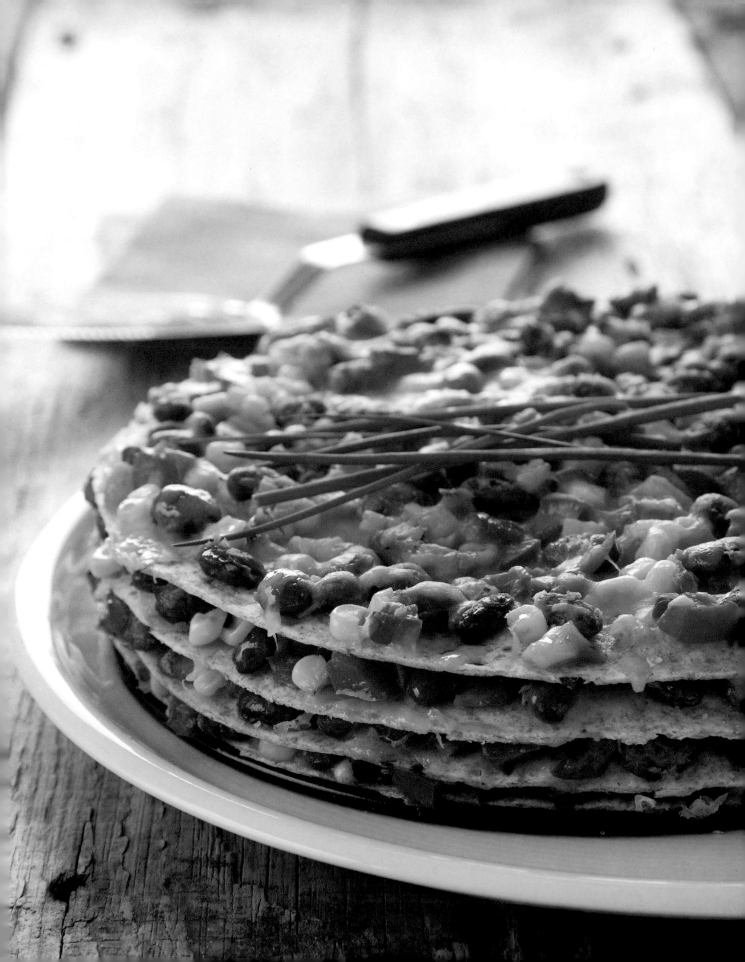

Stacked Tortilla & Bean Pie

This recipe has a spectacular layered presentation and is great for a buffet table. This pie is delicious hot, cold or at room temperature, and it makes great leftovers. —Nettie

1. Preheat the oven to 400°F (200°C). Using a paring knife, trim the tortillas to fit a 9-inch (23 cm) spring-form pan.

2. In a large skillet over medium, heat the oil. Add onion, jalapeno, garlic, cumin, salt and pepper. Cook until softened, about 6 minutes.

3. Add the beans and beer to the skillet, and bring to a boil. Reduce the heat to medium. Simmer until the liquid has evaporated, about 10–12 minutes. Stir in the corn and red pepper. Remove from heat.

4. Place tortilla in bottom of the spring-form pan. Layer with a quarter of the beans and ½ cup (125 mL) cheese. Repeat three more times, finishing with cheese on the top layer.

5. Bake until cheese is melted, about 20 minutes. Unmold the pie; sprinkle with chives. Let stand for 10 minutes to set. Serve sliced into 6 wedges.

Tip: Spring-form pans are not only for cakes! A spring-form pan is ideal for this tortilla pie as it helps to keep the layers intact without the filling falling out. Turn the bottom of the spring-form pan upside down before assembling the pie, since this side of the bottom has no lip, making it easier to slide the pie off after baking.

SERVES 6

4 whole grain tortillas (10 inch/25 cm each), trimmed

1 Tbsp (15 mL) extra virgin olive oil

1 onion, diced

1 jalapeno chile, minced

3 garlic cloves, minced

1 tsp (5 mL) ground cumin

½ tsp (2 mL) sea salt

¼ tsp (1 mL) freshly ground black pepper

19 oz (560 mL) can no-added-salt pinto beans, drained

1¼ cups (300 mL) dark beer or water

1 cup (250 mL) frozen corn niblets

1 red pepper, diced

2 cups (500 mL) shredded cheddar cheese

¼ cup (60 mL) thinly sliced fresh chives

NUTRIENTS PER SERVING SERVING SIZE: ⅙ PIE

415 calories, 18 g fat, 9 g saturated fat, 668 mg sodium, 40 g carbohydrates, 7 g fibre, 4 g sugars, 18 g protein. Very high in fibre. Excellent source of calcium. Good source of riboflavin, folate, vitamin B_{12}, vitamin C, magnesium, and iron.

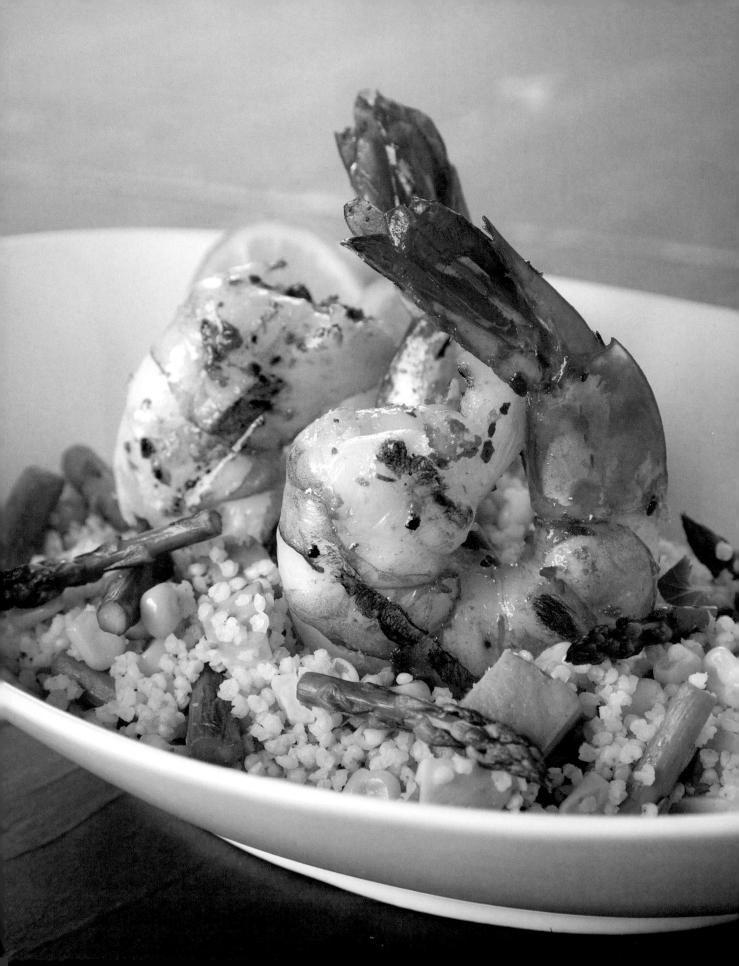

Chili-Lime Shrimp on Millet

If you've never had shrimp made on the barbecue, this recipe is a must-try. Shrimp are simply transformed by barbecue heat, and take on an outer crust with a tender middle. The chili and lime marinade is the perfect combination of spicy and tart, and the fresh cilantro marries all of the ingredients into one cohesive plate. During recipe testing, this dish was my husband, Scott's, favourite. —Cara

1. In a medium-sized bowl, combine the chili flakes, lime zest and 2 Tbsp (30 mL) olive oil. Add the shrimp and stir to coat. Cover and set aside.

2. Heat a medium-sized pot over medium-high heat; add the millet and cook, stirring constantly for 3 minutes until toasted and fragrant.

3. Add water to pot. Reduce the heat to low, cover, and simmer for 20–25 minutes or until the water is absorbed. Remove from the heat and set aside for 10 minutes. Fluff with a fork and transfer to a large bowl.

4. Baste the asparagus with remaining 2 Tbsp (30 mL) oil.

5. Heat a large grill pan or barbecue over high heat. Cook the shrimp for 2 minutes each side or until just cooked through. Set aside.

6. In the pan, cook the asparagus for 5 minutes or until tender-crisp. Slice into 1-inch (2.5 cm) pieces. Add to millet.

7. Add corn, avocado, cilantro and salt to millet. Stir to combine.

8. In a small bowl, whisk together lime juice, oil, chili pepper and sugar. Add to the millet vegetable mixture and toss gently to combine.

9. Divide the millet among serving plates, top with the charred shrimp and serve with lime wedges.

NUTRIENTS PER SERVING SERVING SIZE: ⅙ RECIPE

392 calories, 23 g fat, 3 g saturated fat, 283 mg sodium, 35 g carbohydrates, 7 g fibre, 3 g sugars, 14 g protein. Very high in fibre. Excellent source of vitamin C, vitamin E, vitamin B_{12}, niacin, folate and magnesium. Good source of thiamin, riboflavin, vitamin B_6, iron and zinc.

SERVES 6

½ tsp (2 mL) dried red chili flakes

2 tsp (10 mL) lime zest

¼ cup (60 mL) extra virgin olive oil, divided

1 lb (450 g) frozen shrimp, defrosted, peeled and deveined with tails left intact

1 cup (250 mL) millet

2 cups (500 mL) water

1 bunch asparagus, cut into 1-inch (2.5 cm) pieces

1 cup (250 mL) frozen corn kernels

1 ripe avocado, diced

½ cup (125 mL) coarsely chopped fresh cilantro

½ tsp (2 mL) sea salt

6 lime wedges, to serve

Dressing

3 Tbsp (45 mL) fresh lime juice

3 Tbsp (45 mL) extra virgin olive oil

1 medium red chili pepper, seeded and finely chopped

½ tsp (2 mL) sugar

THE MEDITERRANEAN DIET PYRAMID

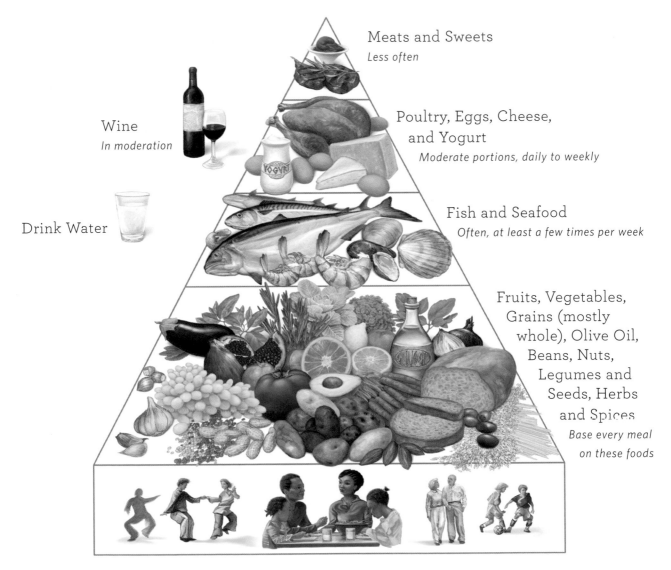

Meats and Sweets
Less often

Wine
In moderation

Poultry, Eggs, Cheese, and Yogurt
Moderate portions, daily to weekly

Drink Water

Fish and Seafood
Often, at least a few times per week

Fruits, Vegetables, Grains (mostly whole), Olive Oil, Beans, Nuts, Legumes and Seeds, Herbs and Spices
Base every meal on these foods

Be Physically Active; Enjoy Meals with Others

Illustration by George Middleton © 2009 Oldways Preservation and Exchange Trust www.oldwayspt.org

A Note About the Mediterranean Diet

The recipes in this book are inspired by foods found in the much-recommended and widely supported Mediterranean diet, which is best represented by this pyramid from Oldways.

The Mediterranean eating plan is a lifestyle, not a diet that you go on for a short time and then abruptly stop. The message in this eating plan is not only about food per se, but about living a healthy lifestyle. It recommends being physically active and sharing meals with others. Cooking is a great way to bring friends and family together around the dinner table. It's not just about what you eat, but where you eat and who you eat with!

THE MEDITERRANEAN DIET

Every meal in the Mediterranean diet, and in our book, is based on these plant-based foods:

Fruits	Legumes (beans, peas and lentils)
Vegetables	Nuts
Whole grains	Seeds
Olive oil	Herbs and spices

The emphasis is on choosing foods that are minimally processed. Animal foods are also included, such as cheese and yogurt, in which small amounts can be eaten every day. Fish, seafood and poultry can be chosen a few times a week, while meat is reserved for a few times a month. At dessert, fruit is the best choice if you crave something sweet, and sugary desserts are left as occasional treats.

The brilliance of this eating plan is in its simplicity. There's no calorie counting, no eliminated food groups, no deprivation from delicious foods. It's just a whole-foods based lifestyle plan that anyone can sustain for optimal wellness.

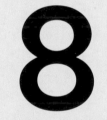

GREEN BEANS WITH PUMPKIN
SEEDS & DILL, P. 174

CHAPTER

8

Vegetable Side Dishes

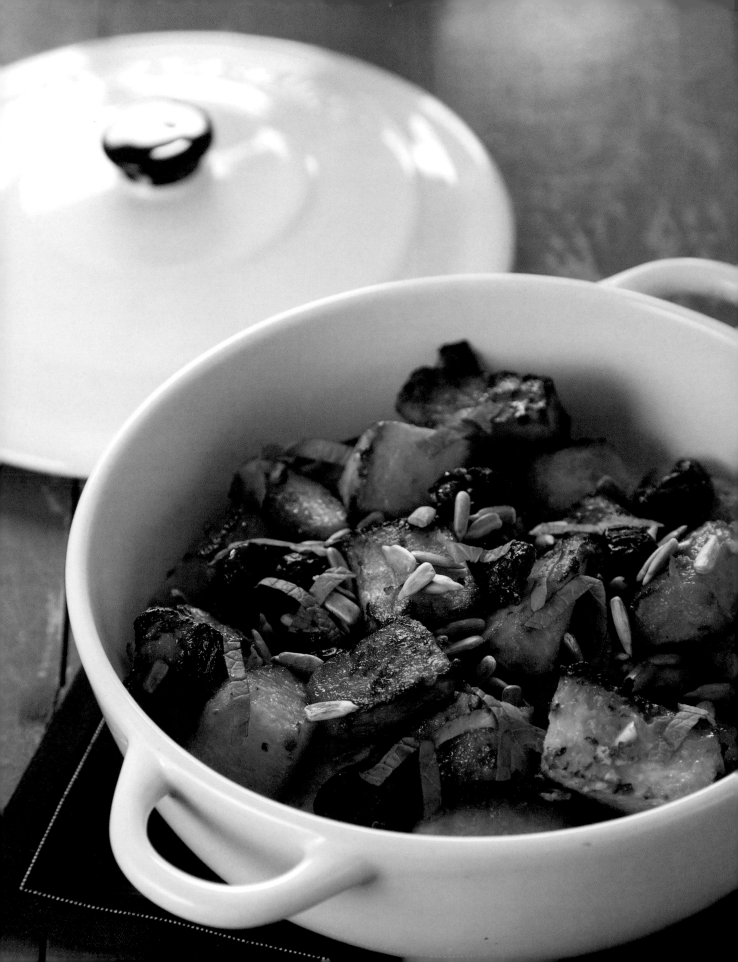

Butternut Squash with Dried Cherries & Mint

Have you ever tried to cut and cube butternut squash? It's not easy! As a simple shortcut, I buy pre-cubed fresh squash, which saves time as the prep work is done for you. The delicate sweetness of squash pairs well with tart cherries and savoury mint. —Cara

1. Preheat oven to 400°F (200°C).
2. In a large bowl, toss butternut squash with oil, garlic, salt and pepper.
3. Transfer squash to a roasting pan or baking dish, and roast until squash is tender and lightly browned, about 30–40 minutes.
4. Top with sunflower seeds, cherries and mint.

 Tip: This recipe also works well with sweet potatoes or acorn squash, instead of butternut.

NUTRIENTS PER SERVING SERVING SIZE: ⅙ RECIPE
98 calories, 3 g fat, 0 g saturated fat, 96 mg sodium, 18 g carbohydrates, 2 g fibre, 7 g sugars, 1 g protein. Excellent source of vitamin A. Good source of vitamin C and magnesium.

SERVES 6

4 cups (1 L) cubed butternut squash

1 Tbsp (15 mL) extra virgin olive oil

1 garlic clove, minced

¼ tsp (1 mL) sea salt

⅛ tsp (0.5 mL) freshly ground black pepper

¼ cup (60 mL) unsalted sunflower seeds, toasted (see page 25)

¼ cup (60 mL) dried tart cherries

¼ cup (60 mL) chopped fresh mint

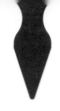

Kale & Red Pepper Stir-Fry

Stir-fries are my favourite side dish. They can accompany so many main courses easily. When buying kale, I look for the smaller, tenderer leaves. They cook quickly and are the tastiest. —Nettie

1. In a large skillet, heat olive oil over medium heat. Add garlic, shallot and ginger. Cook about 3–4 minutes, or until tender.
2. Add the kale and tamari and cook, tossing occasionally until the kale is tender, about 6 minutes. Add red pepper and cook about 4 minutes.
3. Remove from heat into a serving bowl. Add salt, sesame oil and sesame seeds and toss well.

NUTRIENTS PER SERVING SERVING SIZE: ⅙ RECIPE

128 calories, 8 g fat, 1 g saturated fat, 179 mg sodium, 13 g carbohydrates, 3 g fibre, 1 g sugars, 4 g protein. Excellent source of vitamin A and vitamin C. Good source of folate and magnesium.

SERVES 6

2 Tbsp (30 mL) extra virgin olive oil

1 garlic clove, minced

1 shallot, diced

1 tsp (5 mL) grated fresh ginger

8 cups (2 L) chopped kale

1 tsp (5 mL) sodium-reduced tamari

1 red pepper, thinly sliced

¼ tsp (1 mL) sea salt

1 tsp (5 mL) toasted sesame oil

2 Tbsp (30 mL) sesame seeds, toasted (see page 25)

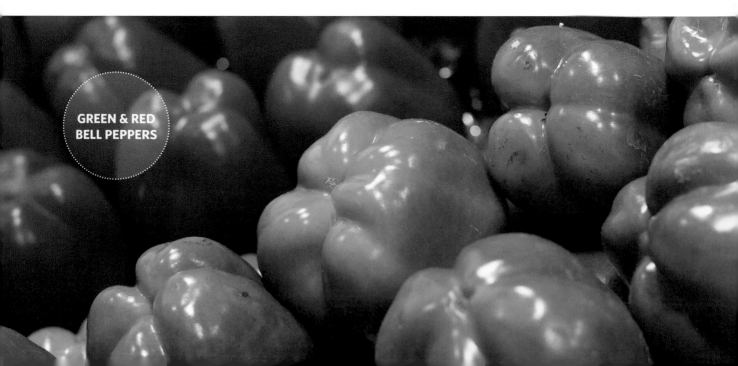

GREEN & RED BELL PEPPERS

Roasted Brussels Sprouts with Tahini Sauce

My friend Robin and I enjoyed a fantastic dinner at Byblos in downtown Toronto. And while everything was excellent, our mutual favourite dish was the Brussels sprouts with tahini. This dish is inspired by that memorable meal. —Cara

1. Preheat oven to 375°F (190°C).
2. In a medium bowl, combine Brussels sprouts, oil, salt and pepper. Transfer mixture to a roasting pan or baking dish. Bake for 35 minutes or until Brussels sprouts are tender and browned.
3. To make the sauce, in a blender, combine tahini, lemon juice, yogurt, water, remaining salt and honey (if using). Blend until combined, about 1 minute. Add more water if sauce is too thick to pour.
4. Pour sauce over Brussels sprouts. Top with sesame seeds.

Tip: Tahini has a bitter taste, which some people love. If you don't, sweeten it a tad with a teaspoon of pure maple syrup or honey.

NUTRIENTS PER SERVING SERVING SIZE: ⅙ RECIPE

77 calories, 5 g fat, 1 g saturated fat, 138 mg sodium, 8 g carbohydrates, 3 g fibre, 2 g sugars, 3 g protein. Excellent source of vitamin C. Good source of folate.

SERVES 6

4 cups (1 L) stemmed and halved Brussels sprouts

1 Tbsp (15 mL) extra virgin olive oil

⅛ tsp (0.5 mL) sea salt

¼ tsp (1 mL) freshly ground black pepper

Sauce

1 Tbsp (15 mL) tahini

2 Tbsp (30 mL) fresh lemon juice

1 Tbsp (15 mL) 2% Greek yogurt

2 Tbsp (30 mL) water

⅛ tsp (0.5 mL) sea salt

1 tsp (5 mL) pure maple syrup or honey (optional)

1 Tbsp (15 mL) sesame seeds, toasted (see page 25)

Green Beans with Pumpkin Seeds & Dill

This recipe has great crunch appeal from the seeds and the lightly steamed green beans. It reminds me of spring. —Nettie

1. Steam green beans for 5 minutes, until tender-crisp.
2. In a large skillet over medium heat, add oil and garlic. Stir in pumpkin seeds and cook until toasted, about 5 minutes.
3. Add steamed green beans, salt, pepper and lemon juice. Stir-fry until coated, about 2 minutes.
4. Transfer to serving bowl and top with fresh dill.

NUTRIENTS PER SERVING SERVING SIZE: ⅙ RECIPE
70 calories, 5 g fat, 1 g saturated fat, 54 mg sodium, 6 g carbohydrates, 2 g fibre, 2 g sugars, 2 g protein.

SERVES 6

4 cups (1 L) green beans

1½ Tbsp (22 mL) extra virgin olive oil

1 garlic clove, minced

2 Tbsp (30 mL) raw unsalted pumpkin seeds

⅛ tsp (0.5 mL) sea salt

⅛ tsp (0.5 mL) freshly ground black pepper

1 Tbsp (15 mL) fresh lemon juice

2 Tbsp (30 mL) chopped fresh dill

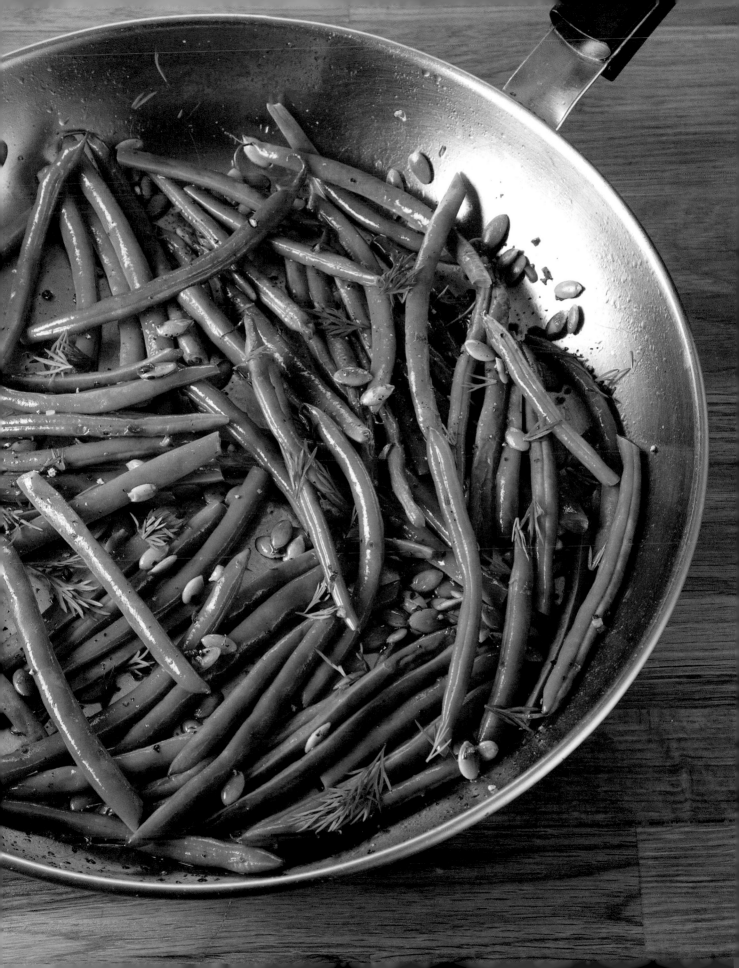

Potatoes with Fresh Herbs

In these lightened-up potatoes, we have replaced the usual cream, butter and salt with fresh herbs, garlic and lemon juice for a delicious dish. They are great at dinner as a side dish! —Nettie

1. Preheat the oven to 400°F (200°C).

2. In a medium-sized bowl, toss potatoes with lemon juice, oil, garlic, salt and pepper.

3. Line a rimmed baking sheet with parchment paper. Spread potatoes onto the baking sheet.

4. Roast for 30 minutes, or until golden brown on the outside and soft in the middle. Stir potatoes halfway through roasting.

5. Add roasted potatoes to a large serving bowl and toss with herbs.

A Note About Potatoes

Potatoes are grown in every province in Canada, with majority hailing from Prince Edward Island. Consumption of these tubers has been on a downward trend, because they are lumped in with the so-called white carbs, which are deemed unhealthy. Deep-fried french fries and chips? Not healthy—true. But skin-on potatoes that are boiled or roasted can be a healthy side dish, to replace pasta, rice or bread. One medium potato with the skin is a good source of vitamin C, potassium and fibre. Of course, portion size is key. Stick with about ½ cup, which is a bit less than one medium-sized potato. In this recipe, 4 potatoes serve 6 people.

SERVES 6

4 medium white potatoes, diced into 1-inch (2.5 cm) squares

1½ Tbsp (22 mL) fresh lemon juice

1 Tbsp (15 mL) extra virgin olive oil

2 garlic cloves, minced

½ tsp (2 mL) sea salt

¼ tsp (1 mL) freshly ground black pepper

2 Tbsp (30 mL) walnuts, toasted (see page 25)

2 Tbsp (30 mL) minced fresh herbs (such as parsley, dill, oregano, chives or cilantro)

NUTRIENTS PER SERVING
SERVING SIZE: ⅙ RECIPE

209 calories, 7 g fat, 1 g saturated fat, 320 mg sodium, 33 g carbohydrates, 4 g fibre, 4 g sugars, 4 g protein. Excellent source of vitamin A. Good source of folate, vitamin C and magnesium.

Broccoli & Cauliflower Stir-Fry with Pecans

Broccoli is reasonably priced, available all year round and easy to prepare. When buying broccoli, look for tightly closed green florets. I like to add cauliflower to this recipe for the colour contrast and complementary texture. Leftovers are delicious cold and can be added to green salads. —Nettie

1. In a skillet over medium heat, add 1½ Tbsp (22 mL) oil and garlic. Cook for 2 minutes.

2. Add broccoli and cauliflower. Stir-fry for about 8–10 minutes, or until tender-crisp; add a teaspoon of water or broth if pan gets too dry or if the garlic starts to brown.

3. Transfer vegetables to a serving bowl; toss with vinegar, remaining oil, salt and pepper; garnish with pecans. Serve family style.

NUTRIENTS PER SERVING SERVING SIZE: ⅙ RECIPE

89 calories, 8 g fat, 1 g saturated fat, 52 mg sodium, 5 g carbohydrates, 2 g fibre, 2 g sugars, 2 g protein. Excellent source of vitamin C. Good source of folate.

SERVES 6

2 Tbsp (30 mL) extra virgin olive oil, divided

1 garlic clove, minced

2 cups (500 mL) broccoli florets, cut into 1½-inch (4 cm) pieces

2 cups (500 mL) cauliflower florets, cut into 1½-inch (4 cm) pieces

2 tsp (10 mL) balsamic vinegar

⅛ tsp (0.5 mL) sea salt

⅛ tsp (0.5 mL) freshly ground black pepper

¼ cup (60 mL) pecan halves, toasted (see page 25)

Marrakesh Cinnamon Vanilla Carrots

This is my son Aubrey's favourite recipe in the book. He calls them "those awesome carrots" as in, "Mom, can you make those awesome carrots again?" Vanilla and cinnamon is such a delicious combination—and I think he loves these because they almost taste like dessert! —Cara

1. In a large frying pan, melt butter over medium heat. Add carrots and sunflower seeds, and stir to combine.

2. Add cinnamon, vanilla, brown sugar and salt. Sauté until carrots are tender-crisp, about 8–10 minutes.

NUTRIENTS PER SERVING SERVING SIZE: ⅙ RECIPE

90 calories, 5 g fat, 3 g saturated fat, 128 mg sodium, 10 g carbohydrates, 3 g fibre, 6 g sugars, 1 g protein. Excellent source of vitamin A.

SERVES 6
2 Tbsp (30 mL) butter
6 carrots, cut into sticks
2 Tbsp (30 mL) sunflower seeds
1 tsp (5 mL) ground cinnamon
1 tsp (5 mL) pure vanilla extract
2 tsp (10 mL) brown sugar
Pinch of sea salt

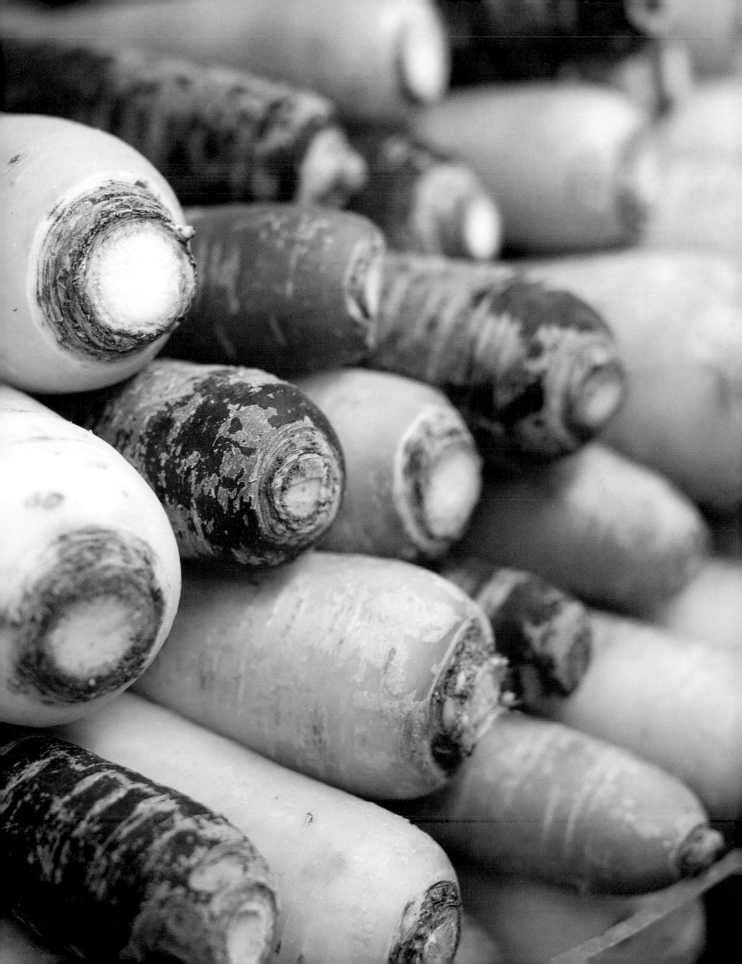

EDAMAME SALAD WITH
CARROT-GINGER DRESSING, P. 79

A Note About Vegetables & Fruit

Vegetables and fruits contain a powerful combination of vitamins, minerals, fibre and antioxidants. These nutrients work together to help you maintain good health and prevent chronic disease.

Each different colour contains unique components that are essential to our health, so fill your plate with a rainbow every day.

Vegetables and fruits are also rich in plant components called phytonutrients, which have beneficial effects on the human body. Many phytonutrients are colour pigments, which give vegetables and fruits their distinctive hues, and many work as antioxidants, which are compounds that may protect cells from changes that lead to heart disease and cancer.

The more colourful your plate is, the greater the variety of nutrients you'll have in your diet. From apricots to zucchinis, enjoy a delicious array of vegetables and fruit to ensure you get all of the helpful, disease-fighting nutrients that your body needs.

PHYTONUTRIENT	COLOUR	BENEFIT
Anthocyanins	Purple: blueberries, cherries, blackberries, red cabbage Red: apples, grapes	May protect against heart disease and help enhance memory, thus preventing age-related declines in mental functioning
Beta-carotene	Orange: carrots, cantaloupe, pumpkin, sweet potato, squash Green: spinach, kale, collards, broccoli	Converts to vitamin A in the body, which plays a role in immune functioning and is critical for normal vision
Lutein	Green: kale, spinach, collards, peas Yellow: corn	Helps reduce risk of cataracts and age-related macular degeneration (the leading cause of blindness in older adults)
Lycopene	Red: tomato, guava, watermelon, papaya, pink grapefruit	May reduce risk of several types of cancer including prostate and breast
Sulfur compounds	White: onion, garlic, leeks, shallots	Has anti-inflammatory, anti-bacterial and anti-viral properties

NUT & SEED BRITTLE, P. 189

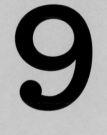

CHAPTER

9

Snacks & Desserts

Peanut Butter Cocoa Bliss Bites

Do you like chocolate truffles? How about peanut butter cups? Now imagine those two were combined into small bites that are best described as "bliss." That's this recipe. My husband, Scott, added a fourth step to this recipe and put the bliss bites in the freezer—he says they are even better that way. Try it for yourself and see which way you prefer them. —Cara

1. In a food processor, combine pumpkin seeds, oats, hemp seeds and sunflower seeds until fine and crumbly, about 1 minute. Add the dates and process for 1 more minute.

2. Add cocoa powder, vanilla, peanut butter and coconut. Process until mixture forms a ball, about 3 minutes.

3. Take small spoonfuls (about 1 Tbsp/15 mL) and roll into 26 bite-sized balls.

Tip: You can dust the bites in powdered sugar, coconut, almond flour or ground nuts for more flavour and texture.

A Note About Dessert

As we discussed the concept of the book, Nettie and I paused when we came the dessert section. How can a healthy cookbook contain 10 desserts? Should we skip that chapter? Or maybe we should prepare low-fat and sugar-free desserts only?

Nope. When you want to eat dessert, it needs to be filled with flavour and sweetness, or it's not really going to be satisfying. Pleasure is an important part of life, and a crucial part of overall health. Typically, enjoying something decadent in moderation won't drastically alter your health or your weight control efforts. But practising portion control is key. And we added some health value to dessert by using ingredients that are both delicious and nutritious, such as coconut, fruit, oats, seeds, nuts and nut butters.

MAKES 26 BITES

½ cup (125 mL) raw unsalted pumpkin seeds

¾ cup (175 mL) large flake rolled oats

⅓ cup (75 mL) hemp seeds

¼ cup (60 mL) raw unsalted sunflower seeds

1½ cups (375 mL) pitted Medjool dates

3 Tbsp (45 mL) cocoa powder

1 tsp (5 mL) pure vanilla extract

½ cup (125 mL) smooth natural peanut butter

2 Tbsp (30 mL) coconut flakes

NUTRIENTS PER SERVING
SERVING SIZE: 1 BITE

98 calories, 5 g fat, 1 g saturated fat, 24 mg sodium, 10 g carbohydrates, 2 g fibre, 6 g sugars, 4 g protein.

Fruit Crisp with Pumpkin Seed Crumble

I will never forget the first time I took my three kids berry picking. Wild blueberry, raspberry and blackberry bushes stretched on for what seemed like miles. My kids wanted to know who to pay and how much the berries would cost! The concept that some food grew wild and one could pick as much as one needed was a valuable lesson for them. We ate as many berries as we could and then made this crisp with the leftover berries. —Nettie

SERVES 12

Filling

4 cups (1 L) mixed berries, hulled

1 apple, peeled and diced

1 pear, peeled and diced

2 Tbsp (30 mL) unsalted butter, melted

1 Tbsp (15 mL) fresh lemon juice

⅛ tsp (0.5 mL) sea salt

½ tsp (2 mL) ground cinnamon

Crumble

½ cup (125 mL) cold unsalted butter

½ cup (125 mL) whole grain wheat flour

¼ cup (60 mL) packed light brown sugar

½ tsp (2 mL) ground cinnamon

¼ tsp (1 mL) sea salt

½ cup (125 mL) large flake rolled oats

½ cup (125 mL) raw unsalted pumpkin seeds

1. Preheat the oven to 350°F (180°C).

2. To make the filling, in a large bowl, combine berries, apple, pear, butter, lemon juice, salt and cinnamon. Stir to combine.

3. In a second bowl, prepare the crumble, combine the butter, flour, sugar, cinnamon and salt. Use a pastry cutter or two forks to mix together until the butter is in small chunks. Stir in the oats and pumpkin seeds.

4. Pour the fruit into a 9 x 13-inch (23 x 33 cm) baking dish. Spread the crumble evenly over top.

5. Bake until the fruit is tender and bubbly and the topping looks solid, about 40–50 minutes.

6. Let cool for 20 minutes; serve warm.

NUTRIENTS PER SERVING SERVING SIZE: ¹/₁₂ RECIPE

202 calories, 13 g fat, 7 g saturated fat, 71 mg sodium, 21 g carbohydrates, 3 g fibre, 11 g sugars, 4 g protein.

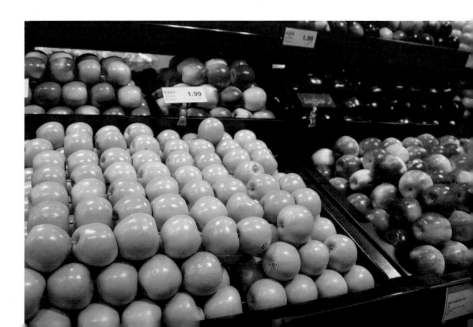

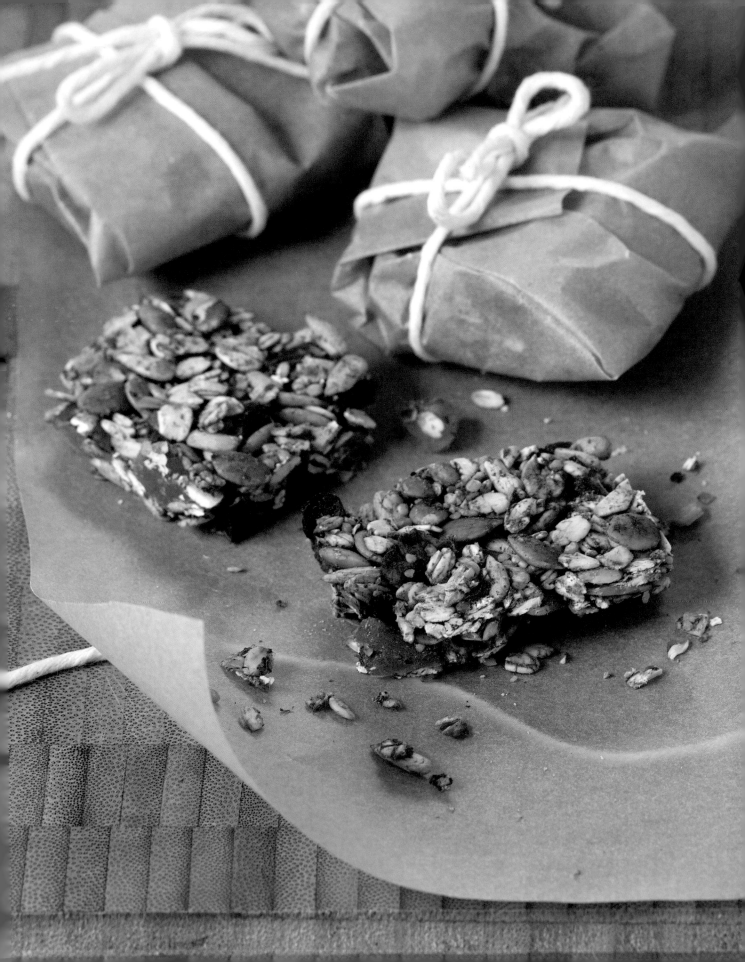

On-the-Go Granola Bars

I have been a hockey mum for 20 years. My current all-star is 15, and he asked me to create his "own" energy bar after buying one and being outraged at the expense. Emery will eat one of these bars 45 minutes before a game and tells me he never fails to set up a goal or score after eating one! —Nettie

1. Preheat the oven to 350°F (180°C). Line a 9 x 13-inch (23 x 33 cm) baking dish with parchment paper.

2. In a large bowl, mash the banana until smooth. Add cinnamon, vanilla, salt, oats and barley flakes and stir well.

3. Add the toasted seeds, coconut, cherries, apricots and dates to the banana-oat mixture and stir until thoroughly combined.

4. Spoon mixture into a baking dish. Press down until compact and even. Bake 25–30 minutes until firm and lightly golden along the edge.

5. Let cool about 10 minutes. Slice into 20 bars.

For tips on toasting seeds, see page 25.

 Tip: These bars can be frozen for 3 months. Wrap individual bars in parchment paper, then aluminum foil. Stack them inside a plastic bag and use a permanent marker to label them.

NUTRIENTS PER SERVING SERVING SIZE: 1 BAR

87 calories, 4 g fat, 1 g saturated fat, 16 mg sodium, 11 g carbohydrates, 2 g fibre, 5 g sugars, 3 g protein.

MAKES 20 BARS

2 ripe bananas, peeled

1 tsp (5 mL) ground cinnamon

½ tsp (2 mL) pure vanilla extract

Pinch of sea salt

½ cup (125 mL) large flaked rolled oats

½ cup (125 mL) barley or oat flakes

½ cup (125 mL) raw unsalted sunflower seeds, toasted

½ cup (125 mL) raw unsalted pumpkin seeds, toasted

¼ cup (60 mL) hemp seeds, toasted

¼ cup (60 mL) unsweetened shredded coconut

¼ cup (60 mL) dried cherries

¼ cup (60 mL) chopped dried apricots

¼ cup (60 mL) pitted and diced Medjool dates

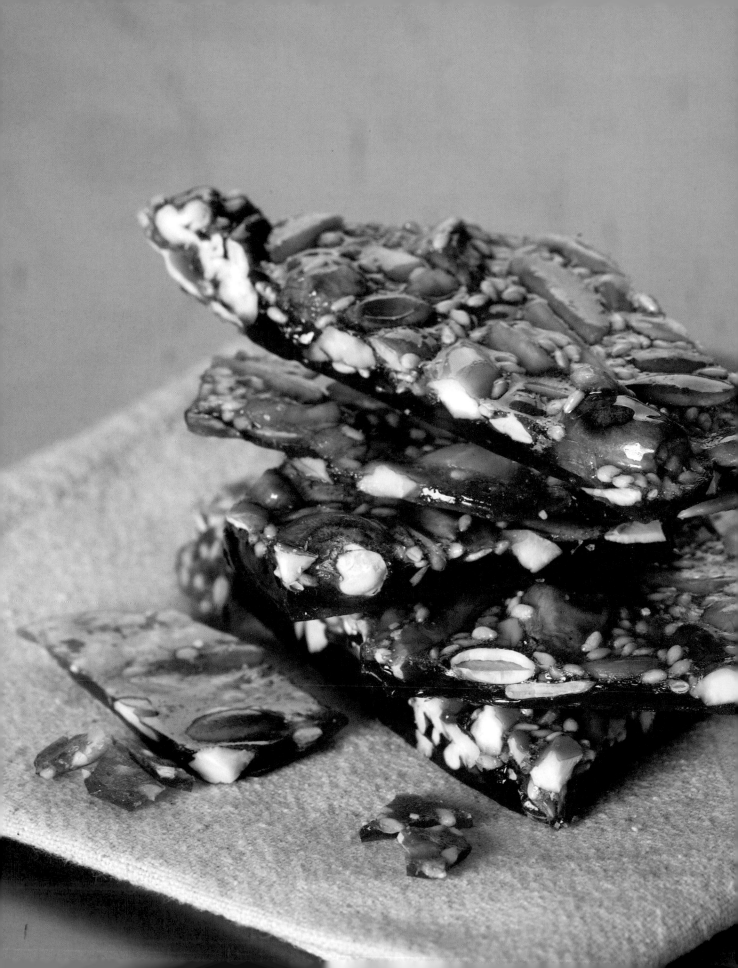

Nut & Seed Brittle

"Why can't we eat the same treats other kids eat?" was a constant refrain in my home as my kids were growing up. As a long-time proponent of healthy eating, I wasn't a big fan of highly processed treats, but I tried my best. My biggest success at candy making was this recipe. Loaded with nuts and seeds, it never lasted past the day it was prepared, and my daughter Macko loved to eat the crumbs. —Nettie

1. Line a 10 x 15-inch (25 x 38 cm) baking sheet with parchment paper. Grease pan with butter. Set aside.

2. Put the sugar in a large saucepan and slowly add the water, taking care not to splash. Stir just to dissolve the sugar, then bring to a simmer over medium-high heat. Let the liquefied sugar simmer until it turns an amber or reddish-brown. Watch it very closely to prevent burning. It should take about 17 minutes. Remove immediately from heat and stir in the remaining ingredients.

3. Pour the mixture onto the prepared baking sheet. Let cool.

4. When brittle is cool, invert to remove from pan. Break into pieces and store in an airtight container.

A Note About Caramelization

Caramelizing is the process of cooking sugar until it browns to a lovely amber colour. Sugar can be caramelized with or without water; using water helps to prevent sugar from burning, making it easier for home cooks like us. After adding the water, stir only once to combine, since stirring lowers the temperature and can delay caramelization. As the sugar darkens in colour, the caramelized flavour gets stronger. Watch the sugar closely as the sugar can go from amber to over-cooked in just a few seconds.

MAKES ABOUT 30 OZ (850 G)

1 Tbsp (15 mL) unsalted butter, softened

2 cups (500 mL) granulated sugar

1 cup (250 mL) water

½ cup (125 mL) sliced almonds

½ cup (125 mL) pecans

½ cup (125 mL) coarsely chopped unsalted pistachios

2 Tbsp (30 mL) raw sesame seeds

2 Tbsp (30 mL) raw unsalted pumpkin seeds

2 Tbsp (30 mL) raw unsalted sunflower seeds

NUTRIENTS PER SERVING
SERVING SIZE: 2 OZ (60 G) BRITTLE

190 calories, 8 g fat, 1 g saturated fat, 2 mg sodium, 29 g carbohydrates, 1 g fibre, 27 g sugars, 2 g protein.

Best-Ever Salted Chocolate Chunk Cookies

This title is no lie. My husband, Scott, is the baker in our household, and these are his absolutely perfect salty-sweet crispy-chewy wonder cookies. I'm a total sucker for chocolate chip cookies, and I share this passion with my niece Jess, who also gives these cookies a big thumbs-up—and that tough cookie is the expert! If you prefer your cookies sweet rather than salty-sweet, you can omit the salt sprinkle. —Cara

1. Preheat oven to 375°F (190°C). Line two baking sheets with parchment paper.

2. In a medium bowl, whisk together flour, baking powder, baking soda and salt. Set aside.

3. Using an electric mixer, beat butter and all sugars on medium speed until light and fluffy, about 4 minutes. Add eggs and vanilla. Beat until mixture is pale and fluffy, about 5 minutes.

4. Using a spatula, slowly add flour mixture, mixing just to blend.

5. Fold in chocolate and Toblerone.

6. Spoon rounded tablespoons of cookie dough onto baking sheets, spacing cookies 1 inch (2.5 cm) apart. Sprinkle cookies with salt.

7. Bake until just golden brown around the edges, 10–12 minutes. Let cool slightly on baking sheets, then transfer to wire racks to cool completely.

NUTRIENTS PER SERVING SERVING SIZE: 1 COOKIE

152 calories, 6 g fat, 4 g saturated fat, 116 mg sodium, 22 g carbohydrates, 1 g fibre, 16 g sugars, 2 g protein.

MAKES 24 COOKIES

1½ cups (500 mL) all-purpose flour

1 tsp (5 mL) baking powder

¼ tsp (1 mL) baking soda

¼ tsp (1 mL) sea salt

½ cup (125 mL) unsalted butter, room temperature

¾ cup (175 mL) packed light brown sugar

½ cup (125 mL) granulated sugar

¼ cup (60 mL) icing sugar

2 large eggs

1 tsp (5 mL) pure vanilla extract

½ cup (125 mL) semi-sweet chocolate, coarsely chopped

½ cup (125 mL) Toblerone, coarsely chopped

2 Tbsp (30 mL) ground flaxseeds

1 tsp (5 mL) Maldon or kosher salt (optional)

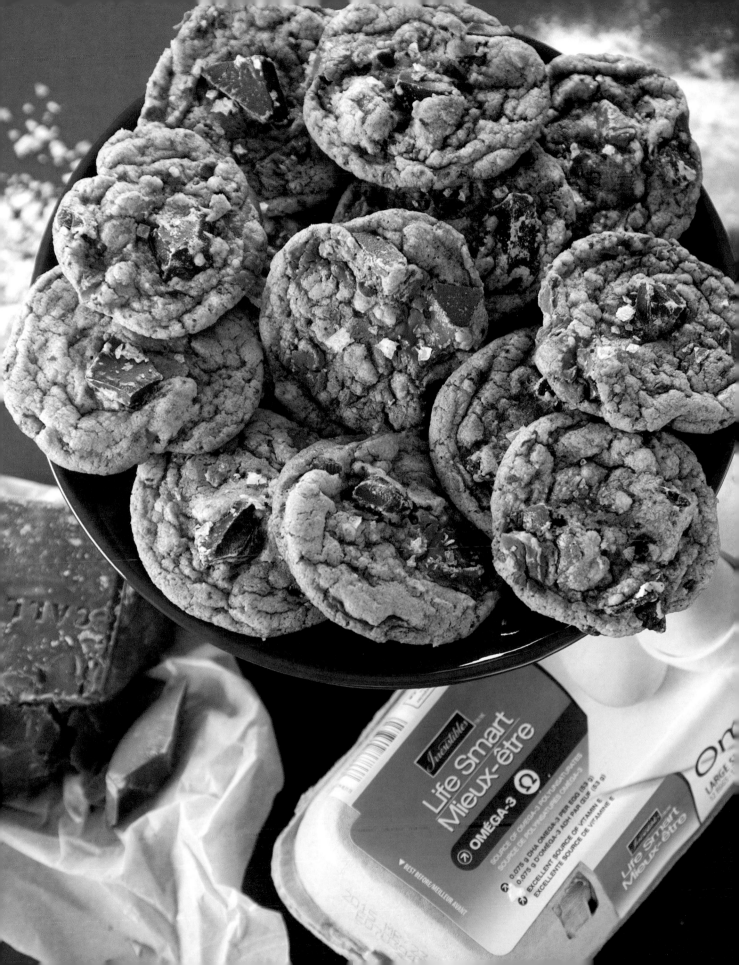

Banana Oat Muffins

These muffins are a staple in my house—particularly in my freezer. My kids and I make a batch any time we have ripe bananas, enjoy one each and freeze the leftovers. They make perfect recess snacks. If you prefer, you can also use 2% Greek yogurt instead of the ricotta cheese. And of course, chocolate chips are a great addition too! —Cara

1. Preheat oven to 350°F (180°C). Line a 12-cup muffin pan with paper liners.
2. In a medium bowl, whisk together bananas, brown sugar, ricotta, oil and egg.
3. In a large bowl, whisk together flours, oats, flaxseed, chia seeds, baking soda, baking powder, cinnamon and vanilla.
4. Add wet mixture and flour mixture and stir just until blended; do not over-mix.
5. Spoon batter into prepared muffin pan. Bake for 18-20 minutes, or until tops are firm to the touch and a tester inserted into the centre of a muffin comes out clean.

Tip: If you don't have ripe bananas, you can use two ½ cup (125 mL) jars of banana baby food. Or, one ripe banana and one jar of baby food. To mix it up, you can also replace one of the bananas (or ½ cup) with puréed pumpkin, sweet potato, mango, apple or any other baby food!

MAKES 12 MUFFINS

2 medium ripe bananas, mashed

½ cup (125 mL) packed brown sugar

⅓ cup (75 mL) ricotta cheese

3 Tbsp (45 mL) canola oil

1 large egg

1 cup (250 mL) whole oat flour

½ cup (125 mL) whole barley flour

½ cup (125 mL) large flake rolled oats

¼ cup (60 mL) ground flaxseeds

1 Tbsp (15 mL) chia seeds

1 tsp (5 mL) baking soda

1 tsp (5 mL) baking powder

½ tsp (2 mL) ground cinnamon

1 tsp (5 mL) pure vanilla extract

NUTRIENTS PER SERVING
SERVING SIZE: 1 MUFFIN

202 calories, 7 g fat, 1 g saturated fat, 145 mg sodium, 30 g carbohydrates, 3 g fibre, 12 g sugars, 5 g protein.

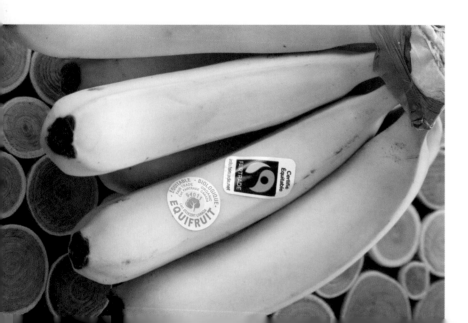

Millet Oatmeal Raisin Cookies

Like most kids, my children love to eat cookies. Rather than buy store-bought, we'll bake together and create cookies with better-for-you ingredients. These crunchy cookies contain millet, oats, sunflower seeds, raisins and whole grain flours—but to my kids, they are just cookies! The time spent baking them together makes them taste even better. —Cara

MAKES 24 COOKIES

1 cup (250 mL) whole grain wheat flour

¼ cup (60 mL) oat flour

¾ cup (175 mL) large flake rolled oats

⅓ cup (75 mL) millet

½ tsp (2 mL) baking soda

½ tsp (2 mL) baking powder

1 tsp (5 mL) ground cinnamon

¼ tsp (1 mL) ground nutmeg

¼ tsp (1 mL) ground ginger

¼ tsp (1 mL) sea salt

½ cup (125 mL) unsalted butter, melted

½ cup (125 mL) pure maple syrup

2 large eggs, beaten

1 tsp (5 mL) pure vanilla extract

⅓ cup (75 mL) raisins

⅔ cup (150 mL) unsalted sunflower seeds, toasted (see page 25)

1. Preheat oven to 350°F (180°C). Line two baking sheets with parchment paper.

2. In a large bowl, whisk together whole grain flour, oat flour, oats, millet, baking soda, baking powder, cinnamon, nutmeg, ginger and salt.

3. In another large bowl, whisk together the butter, maple syrup, eggs and vanilla. Add to the flour mixture and stir until combined.

4. Stir in the raisins and sunflower seeds.

5. Let the dough rest for 10 minutes, to thicken slightly.

6. Spoon rounded tablespoons of cookie dough onto baking sheets. Gently flatten cookies. Space them 1 inch (2.5 cm) apart.

7. Bake for about 14 minutes. Transfer to a rack to cool completely.

NUTRIENTS PER SERVING SERVING SIZE: 1 COOKIE

119 calories, 5 g fat, 3 g saturated fat, 61 mg sodium, 15 g carbohydrates, 1 g fibre, 6 g sugars, 3 g protein.

Tip: Buy assorted cheeses to accompany the Date & Fig Slices and serve them with Sunflower Barley Crackers, page 75.

Date & Fig Slices

I do not consider myself to be a "food snob," but my husband, Jim, begs to differ! He likes to remind me of the time he bought the wrong type of fig and date for this recipe. So, to keep the record straight, the best types to buy are Medjool dates and Mission figs. Medjool dates impart a deep, complex flavour, reminiscent of chocolate. Mission figs are sweet and fleshy with a soft skin and delicate tiny seeds. The paste they make is exquisite. This recipe is best served with an assortment of sharp cheeses and specialty crackers. —Nettie

1. In the bowl of a food processor, combine oats, hazelnuts, coconut, chia seeds, cinnamon, cardamom, cocoa and vanilla. Process for 3 minutes or until ingredients are well combined.

2. With the motor running, start adding the dates and figs, a few pieces at a time, processing until all have been added and the mixture is sticking together. Add orange juice and lemon zest. Mix well.

3. Transfer date and fig paste to a sheet of parchment paper. Shape it into a rough 10-inch (25 cm) log, then wrap it tightly and add a sheet of aluminium foil on top of the parchment paper to shape it into a cylinder. Refrigerate for 1 hour.

4. Slice into 16 pieces and serve cold or at room temperature.

MAKES 16 SLICES

1½ cups (500 mL) large flake rolled oats

½ cup (125 mL) raw unsalted hazelnuts

¼ cup (60 mL) shredded coconut

¼ cup (60 mL) chia seeds

½ tsp (2 mL) ground cinnamon

¼ tsp (1 mL) ground cardamom

1½ Tbsp (22 mL) cocoa powder

2 tsp (10 mL) pure vanilla extract

1½ cups (500 mL) chopped and pitted dates

1 cup (250 mL) stemmed and halved dried figs

1 Tbsp (15 mL) orange juice

½ tsp (2 mL) lemon zest

Tip: Many recipes require lemon, lime or orange zest, which is the thin layer of peel that contains flavourful citrus oil. When making zest, look for organic citrus fruits, since the rind on conventionally grown fruits can retain pesticide residue.

NUTRIENTS PER SERVING SERVING SIZE: 1 SLICE

155 calories, 4 g fat, 0 g saturated fat, 3 mg sodium, 30 g carbohydrates, 5 g fibre, 18 g sugars, 3 g protein. High in fibre.

Maple-Chipotle Popcorn

Stove-top popcorn is a snacking staple in my house. My husband, Scott, is the resident popcorn master, as our guests can attest to. It's always on offer. On special occasions he'll make his famous caramel corn, or this spicier, maple-based version. We shy away from microwave popcorn, since fat, salt and preservatives may be added. Plus, making it on the stovetop or in an air popper is much more fun! —Cara

1. Preheat the oven to 350°F (180°C).

2. Line two rimmed baking sheet with foil.

3. Lightly coat one baking sheet and a wooden spoon with 1 Tbsp (15 mL) canola oil.

4. In a large saucepan with a lid, heat the remaining 3 Tbsp (45mL) canola oil over medium-high heat. Add the popcorn kernels, cover and cook, shaking the pan occasionally to prevent burning. When the popping slows to 3–5 seconds between pops, remove from the heat and let cool for 5 minutes. Transfer to a large bowl and remove unpopped kernels.

5. On the foil-lined baking sheet without canola oil, spread the pecans and sunflower seeds in a single layer. Bake for 7–8 minutes, until lightly toasted and fragrant. When cool enough to handle, coarsely chop. Add to popcorn and toss to combine.

6. In a small saucepan, melt the butter over medium heat. Stir in the maple syrup, ground chili and salt, then bring to a boil and cook, without stirring, until the mixture reaches 300°F (150°C) on a candy thermometer, about 15–20 minutes.

7. Pour the syrup over the popcorn and quickly stir with the oiled spoon to evenly coat. Immediately spread the mixture on the foil-lined and oiled pan. Let cool completely, and then break into bite-sized pieces and serve.

8. Store leftovers in an airtight container at room temperature for up to 3 days.

SERVES 10

4 Tbsp canola oil, divided

⅓ cup (75 mL) popcorn kernels

½ cup (125 mL) raw pecans

½ cup (125 mL) raw unsalted sunflower seeds

6 Tbsp (90 mL) unsalted butter

1½ cups (375 mL) pure maple syrup

½ tsp (2 mL) ground chipotle chili powder

½ tsp (2 mL) sea salt

NUTRIENTS PER SERVING
SERVING SIZE: 1 CUP (250 ML) POPCORN

263 calories, 15 g fat, 5 g saturated fat, 93 mg sodium, 33 g carbohydrates, 2 g fibre, 24 g sugars, 2 g protein.

Multi-Grain Scones

These scones are equally great at breakfast, tea time or dessert. They freeze well too. —Cara

1. Preheat oven to 375°F (190°C).
2. In a medium-sized bowl, whisk the egg, sugar, milk, oil and lemon zest together.
3. In a separate large bowl, mix together the oats, wheat bran, flour, cherries, hemp seeds, millet, poppy seeds, salt, baking powder and cinnamon. Stir with a wooden spoon.
4. Add wet mixture to dry mixture to create a thick dough.
5. Drop 12 spoonfuls of batter onto a baking sheet lined parchment paper. Bake for 15–20 minutes, just until golden. Remove from the oven and let cool.

Tip: If you can't find dried cherries, you can use dried cranberries instead.

A Note About Flour

Whole wheat flour is not a whole grain. That sounds crazy, but in Canada, whole wheat flour is processed to preserve shelf life. When that happens, about 5 percent of the kernel is removed—the most nutirent-dense parts that contain most of the germ and some of the bran. When removed, most of the fibre, vitamins and minerals are removed too. Instead of whole wheat flour, look for 100 percent whole grain wheat flour—try the one by Rogers, Bob's Red Mill or Oak Manor. You can also makes these amazing scones with whole spelt flour.

MAKES 12 SCONES

1 large egg

¼ cup (60 mL) granulated sugar

½ cup (125 mL) 2% milk

5 Tbsp (75 mL) canola oil

1 Tbsp (15 mL) lemon zest

½ cup (125 mL) large-flake rolled oats

¼ cup (60 mL) wheat bran

1 ½ cups (500 mL) whole grain wheat flour

¼ cup (60 mL) chopped dried cherries

2 Tbsp (30 mL) hemp seeds, toasted (see page 25)

2 Tbsp (30 mL) millet

2 Tbsp (30 mL) poppy seeds

½ tsp (2 mL) sea salt

1 Tbsp (15 mL) baking powder

½ tsp (2 mL) cinnamon

NUTRIENTS PER SERVING
SERVING SIZE: 1 SCONE

186 calories, 8 g fat, 1 g saturated fat, 182 mg sodium, 24 g carbohydrates, 3 g fibre, 7 g sugars, 4 g protein.

A Note About Sugar

Sugar is found in many foods; sometimes it occurs naturally, and sometimes it is added.

Natural sugars are found in fruit, milk and sweet-tasting vegetables, such as beets and sweet potatoes.

Added sugars are used in food manufacturing to make foods taste sweet. While sugar is obviously added to foods such as pop and candy, it's also used in surprising places, like barbeque sauce and crackers.

Natural and added sugars aren't exactly equal, and here's why: foods like vegetables and fruit with natural sugars also contain fibre, vitamins and minerals that provide essential nutrients to the body. So, while a kiwi may have 7 grams of sugar, it also contains fibre and vitamin C. On the other hand, 10 small jellybeans also contain 7 grams of sugar. But that's it. They contain nothing else. No fibre. No vitamins. Clearly the kiwi is the better choice for the same amount of sugar.

Sugar that's added to food products may be listed as brown sugar, honey, maple syrup, coconut sugar, agave, evaporated cane juice, granulated sugar or a dozen other names. Remember, they are all sugar, and provide little more than calories. They are not nutrient-dense.

Studies show that excess sugar consumption is associated with heart disease, stroke, obesity, diabetes, high blood cholesterol and some types of cancer. What is excess consumption? Twelve teaspoons of added sugar in a day. Note: these numbers are for added sugars, not for natural sugars in fruit and milk.

People with intakes above 12 teaspoons (50 g) of added sugar in a day have a 30 percent higher risk of death from heart disease or stroke when compared to those who consume less than 10 percent—that's why that cut-off of a maximum of 12 teaspoons (50 g) per day was established. For those who consume 25 percent or more of calories from added sugar, the risk of heart disease is nearly tripled.

So, as a dietitian, here are my five key points for sugar guidance:

1. Don't deny yourself desserts once in a while, but keep the portions small.

2. If you crave sweets, choose fruit, dried fruit or other naturally sweet foods that also have some nutritional value.

3. Keep your intake of added sugars low—no more than 12 teaspoons (50 g) per day as a maximum. Less, of course, is better.

4. Added sugars are found in almost all processed foods and drinks, so read nutrition labels carefully and choose foods with less sugar.

5. The easiest way to cut back on sugar is to stop drinking pop. A 12 oz (355mL) can of pop contains about 10 teaspoons (40 grams) of sugar and has no health benefits.

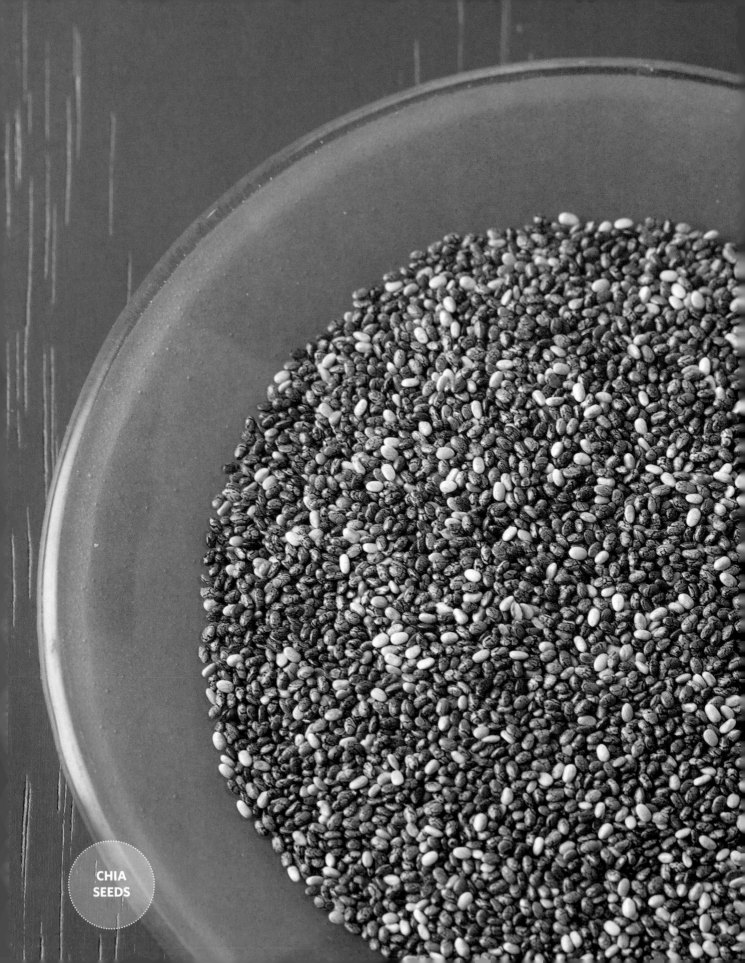

CHIA
SEEDS

Glossary

APPLE CIDER VINEGAR: This is an inexpensive, fruity tasting vinegar that needs refrigeration if unpasteurized. Its low level of acidity allows it to contribute flavour without overwhelming other ingredients, especially in salad dressing.

ARAME: Arame is an edible sea vegetable (a name that is superior to seaweed) gathered from the ocean that is sold dried, cut and packaged. It's reconstituted by adding water or stock and soaking for 5 minutes. It resembles black angel hair pasta and can be used in soups, salads and casseroles.

ARUGULA: A salad green, arugula is often added to the salad mix known as mesclun because of its peppery taste. It is related to the radish, and may also be called rocket.

BALSAMIC GLAZE: This is a thick, syrupy reduction of balsamic vinegar. It is sold as balsamic glaze, syrup or reduction. You can also make your own by putting balsamic vinegar in a saucepan over medium heat and reducing it by half.

BALSAMIC VINEGAR: Made from sweet Trebbiano grapes (skins and juice) that are crushed and fermented in wooden casks in the Italian region of Emilia-Romagna, near the town of Modena. The mellow sweet-tart flavour best suits vinaigrette salad dressings or splashed on steamed or grilled ingredients.

BARLEY FLOUR: Barley flour is milled from barley and can be used in recipes such as bread, cakes and cookies. Be sure to choose whole grain barley flour, which contains all parts of the barley kernel—the germ, endosperm and bran. Barley flour has a sweet, nut-like flavour.

BROWN RICE VINEGAR: A mildly sweet vinegar made from fermented brown rice. Used extensively in Japanese and Chinese cuisine, rice vinegar enhances the flavour of plain rice. It is good in salad dressings and soy-based dips and sauces. It can be used as a pickling ingredient as well. When traditionally brewed, unfiltered rice vinegars often contain rice sediment that can make the liquid look cloudy, but this is a sign of good quality.

BUCKWHEAT: Buckwheat is not related to wheat at all; buckwheat is a plant that's part of the rhubarb family and is used as a culinary whole grain. It has a strong, earthy flavour and cooks quickly in water (about 15 minutes). One way to keep the individual grains intact during cooking is to toast them first.

BROWN SUGAR: Brown sugar is refined white sugar with molasses added. It is available in light and dark varieties. The darker the colour, the more intense the flavour.

CAPERS: Capers are the flower buds of a Mediterranean shrub. They are pickled and used as a salty, briny condiment.

CARDAMOM: Grown in many parts of India,

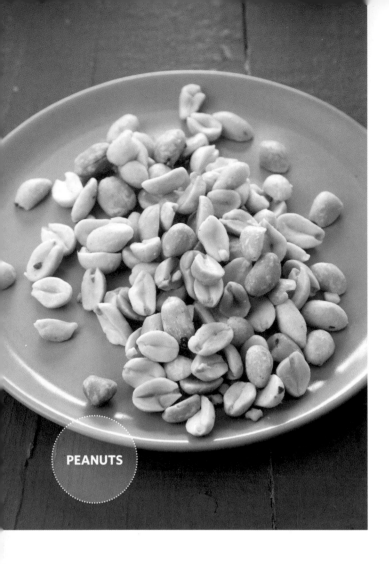

PEANUTS

Mexico and South America, cardamom is a spice that's used in the sweet and savoury dishes of many cuisines. Both whole pods and ground cardamom are available. It has a complex, sweet-spicy flavour and aroma.

CHILI PEPPERS: Chilies are available in many forms—fresh, dried, ground or canned. The heat is in the ribs and membranes that hold the seeds. Their volatile oils can cause a lot of discomfort if you touch your mouth or eyes after handling. You can protect yourself by wearing thin rubber gloves. Always wash your hands after handling chilies.

CILANTRO: Cilantro is a leafy green herb with a distinct and hard-to-describe flavour that is quite polarizing—you either love it or can't stand it! Cilantro is sometimes called coriander when you buy the fresh herb, but usually coriander refers to the dried seed or ground spice, and cilantro refers to the fresh leafy herbs. They are all part of the same plant, though.

COCONUT MILK: Made by soaking shredded fresh coconut in hot water. When using canned coconut milk, make sure you mix the thin liquid at the top with the bottom, creamy thick layer. Refrigerate leftover milk for a maximum of 3 days.

COCONUT OIL: This is the fatty oil obtained from coconuts. It can be used as a replacement for butter or margarine in recipes. If used when stir-frying or deep frying, the ingredients will not absorb the oil.

CUMIN: Cumin seeds are the dried fruit of the cumin plant. Whole seeds and ground are available. Cumin is often a part of another spice mixture, such as curry or garam masala, but it can also be used on its own. Lightly toasting the seeds before grinding enhances their flavour.

FENNEL: This is a crunchy bulbous vegetable with stalks and fuzzy fronds attached, and a slightly anise/black licorice flavour. Peel off the outer membrane and the root end before using them. Serve fennel raw, thinly sliced, shaved or braised in stock.

GARAM MASALA: Garam masala is the classic ground spice blend of Northern India. You can make it yourself or buy a ready-made spice blend. It contains any combination of cardamom, cinnamon, cumin, cloves, coriander, black peppercorns and nutmeg.

GREEK YOGURT: This is a thick, creamy yogurt that has been double-strained. It contains double the protein and half the carbohydrates when compared to regular yogurt.

HALLOUMI CHEESE: Popular in Greece and Cyprus, this semi-hard cheese is unique because it has a high melting point, so it can be fried or grilled.

KOMBU: Kombu is a sea vegetable often used as part of a soup and stock base. A strip of kombu cooked with water releases glutamic acid (a white powdery coating which contains a lot of flavour). Do not rinse it off before cooking. Glutamic acid is the natural version of that synthetic flavouring agent monosodium glutamate (MSG).

LARGE-FLAKE ROLLED OATS: These are oat groats that have been heated to soften them, and then rolled flat. They are a natural whole grain and can be used to make oatmeal, and are excellent for baking.

MAPLE SYRUP: This is a sweet syrup made from boiling the spring sap tapped from sugar maple trees. It is graded according to colour, flavour and sugar content, maple syrups with a B or C designation can be used for baking and cooking. Grade A syrup is lighter, more delicate and is best used as a topping for pancakes and ice cream.

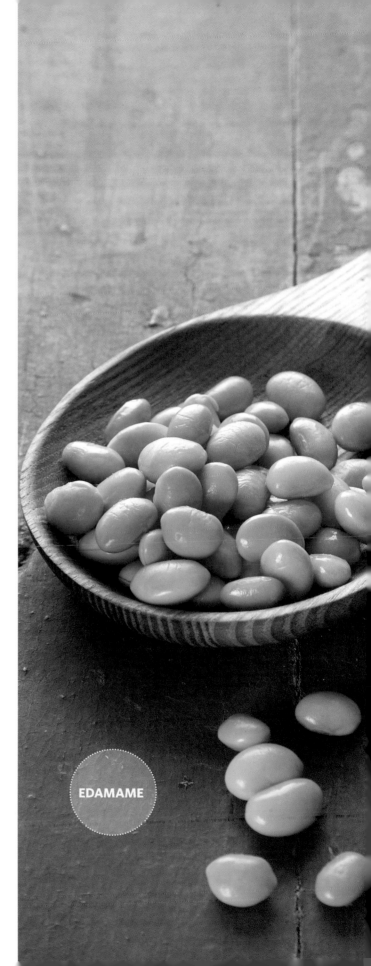

EDAMAME

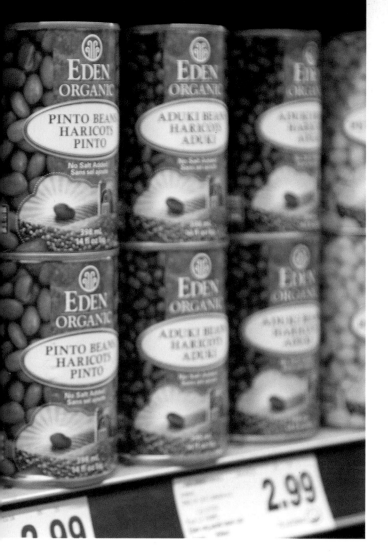

2.99

MEDJOOL DATES: These are large, sweet and plump dates, with a moist thick flesh. They are high in potassium and fibre.

MIRIN: Mirin is a sweet rice wine used in Japanese cooking. It can be used to balance the saltiness of other seasonings like miso and soy sauce or in sauces, glazes and vinaigrettes. Mirin is made from water, sweet brown rice and rice culture.

MISO: Miso is to vegetarian cooking what beef bouillon or gravy is to a meat-centred diet. This salty, fermented paste is made from aged soybeans and grains. Thick and spreadable, it is used for flavouring in a wide variety of recipes and for being the basic ingredient in many soups. It's available in the refrigerated section of your local health food store and comes in several varieties. Some grocery stores carry miso as well. Dark miso tends to be saltier and have a stronger flavour than lighter varieties. Shiro, or white miso, has a pale yellow colour and a mild taste. Miso will keep for 6 months when refrigerated in an airtight container.

NORI: This is a sea vegetable that has been dried and pressed into sheets. Used for wrapping sushi rolls and also as a garnish when cut into thin strips or shredded. Available at most grocery stores in the sushi or ethnic foods section, it is sold in sheets.

OAT FLOUR: Oat flour is finely milled oat groats. Oats are harvested with their hulls intact. Remove the hull and the remaining grain is an oat groat. If you cannot find oat flour, simply grind up large-flake rolled oats in a blender or spice grinder.

OLIVE OIL: Olive oil is pressed from olives. Extra virgin olive oil is the first pressing of the olive. Buy a good quality olive oil, packaged in dark coloured glass to protect it from sunlight. Look for olive oil with a best before date—it does not get better with age and can go rancid quite readily.

SOBA NOODLES: Long, thin Japanese noodles

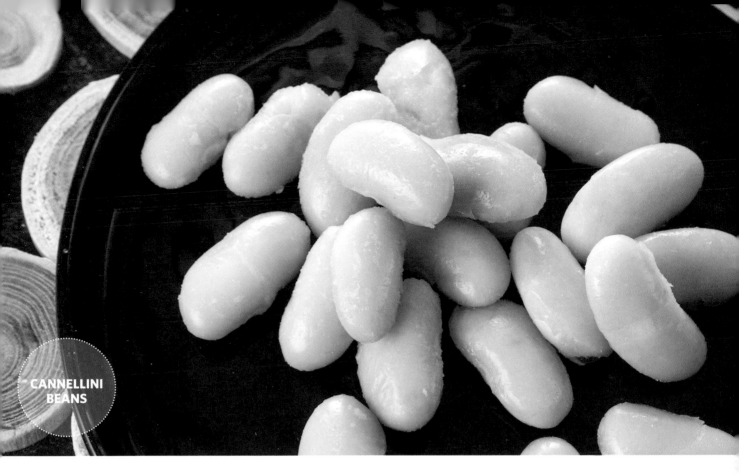

CANNELLINI
BEANS

made from 100 percent buckwheat flour or a combination of buckwheat and unbleached or whole wheat flours. Soba comes in several varieties with varying percentages of buckwheat; other ingredients can be added for extra flavour. These noodles are eggless and less sticky than Italian pasta.

SPELT FLOUR: Spelt, a strain of wheat, is one of the ancient grains. It has a texture similar to standard wheat. It can be substituted for whole wheat flour. Look for whole grain spelt flour for the best nutritional value.

STEEL-CUT OATS: Steel-cut oats are also called Irish oats. They are made from oat groats that have been cut horizontally with a heavy steel blade. They require an overnight soaking or lengthy cooking to be eaten. They take longer to cook than large flake oats, don't cook down as much and have a chewier consistency.

TAHINI: This is a thick, smooth paste made of hulled and ground sesame seeds. A Middle Eastern staple, tahini is used as a spread and as an ingredient in dressings, sauces and dips.

TAMARI: Tamari is type of soy sauce that's made with no (or very little) wheat, while traditional soy sauce does contain wheat. It's very salty, so we use a sodium-reduced version.

TOASTED SESAME OIL: Oil made from toasted sesame seeds. Darker in colour than plain sesame oil with a wonderful aroma and a toasty, nutty flavour. It is not to be confused with sesame oil, which has a milder, less distinct flavour. They are not interchangeable.

WASABI POWDER: Wasabi is a light green Japanese root vegetable that is very hot, with a taste reminiscent of horseradish. It is sold dried and powdered. For cooking or serving as a condiment, the powder is mixed with water and made into a paste.

Details About
Nutrient Analysis

The nutrient analysis for the recipes was completed by Amy Whitson, PHEc, from The Test Kitchen Incorporated. She used NutriBase Professional Edition software, which uses information sourced from the Canadian Nutrient File, USDA Nutrient Database for Standard Reference and Nutrition Facts information from consumer product labels. The nutritional content claims are based on the criteria established by the Canadian Food Inspection Agency's Nutrition Labelling regulations. When a recipe serving provides at least 25 percent of the Daily Recommended Intake (DRI) of a vitamin or mineral, it is considered an Excellent Source; if a recipe serving provides 15 percent of the DRI, it is considered a Good Source.

Recipe analysis is based on one serving, as indicated for each recipe where it says "serving size." Optional ingredients are not included in nutrient analysis. For example, recipe analysis for Quinoa and Berry Hot Cereal does not include the honey or Greek yogurt, which are optional ingredients.

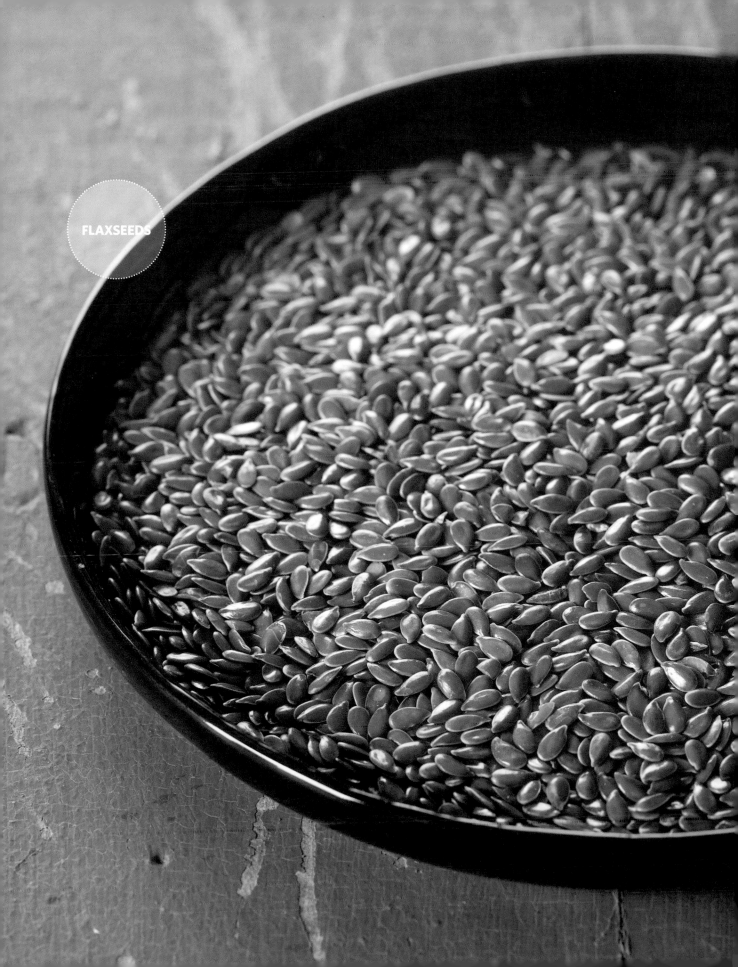

FLAXSEEDS

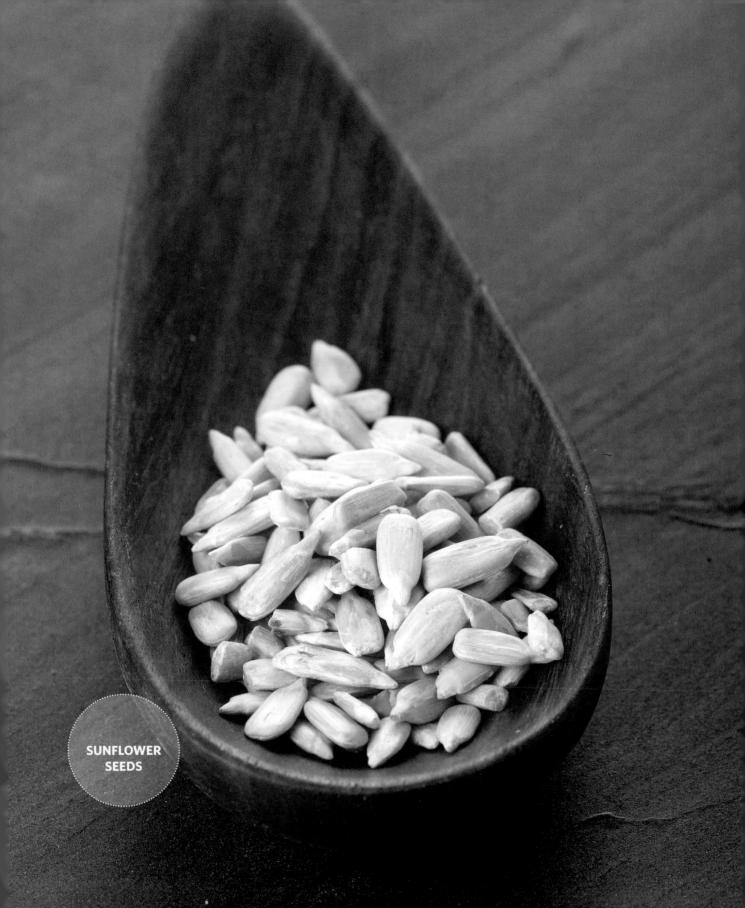

SUNFLOWER
SEEDS

For Further Reading

To learn more about the connection between healthy eating, whole foods and disease prevention, here are some further resources to read:

Helpful diet and nutrition advice. **EatRight Ontario:** *www.eatrightontario.ca*

Mediterranean Diet. **Oldways:** *www.oldwayspt.org/resources/heritage-pyramids/mediterranean-diet-pyramid*

Position statement: Sugar, heart disease and stroke. **Heart and Stroke Foundation:** *www.heartundstroke.com/site/c.iklQLcMWJtE/b.9201361/k.47CB/Sugar_heart_disease_and_stroke.htm*

Your Guide to Lowering Blood Pressure. National Heart, Lung, and Blood Institute. **US Department of Health and Human Services:** *www.nhlbi.nih.gov/files/docs/public/heart/hbp_low.pdf*

Diet for diabetes. **American Diabetes Association:** *www.diabetes.org/food-and-fitness/food/planning-meals/diabetes-meal-plans-and-a-healthy-diet.html*

Your Guide to Lowering Your Cholesterol with TLC. **National Heart, Lung, and Blood Institute. US Department of Health and Human Services:** *www.nhlbi.nih.gov/files/docs/public/heart/chol_tlc.pdf.*

Advice from registered dietitians: *www.dietitians.ca*

What We Used

We tested recipes using exceptional products, and we wish to thank all of the fine companies that supported the recipe development and photography for this book.

Blendtec provided us with the Blendtec Designer 725, a great blender for recipe testing. It is exceptionally powerful, and really helped with the texture of our soups, salad dressings, dips and smoothie recipes. Thank you to Sarah Guffey. *www.blendtec.com*

Breville generously donated their "Fastest Slow Cooker" so we could test our made-from-scratch bean cooking times. It's both a slow cooker and a pressure cooker. *www.breville.ca*

Campbell's Company of Canada donated countless litres of their Campbell's No-Salt-Added Vegetable Broth, which was used for testing appetizers, soups and entrées. It was an easy way to make lower sodium soups, since it contains just 33 mg of sodium per cup. Thanks to Teresa Mastrodicasa RD. *www.campbellsoup.ca*

Catelli provided the pasta that we used for recipe testing. We used Catelli Healthy Harvest 100 percent whole grain spaghetti and penne, made from whole grain durum semolina. We also used Healthy Harvest multigrain fusilli, which is made with a blend of whole grain wheat, rye, buckwheat, barley and brown rice. Thanks to Gail Bergman. *www.catelli.ca*

Central Roast provided a variety of nuts and seeds including almonds, pecans, pumpkin seeds and pine nuts. Thanks to John Hopperton. *www.centralroastbrands.com*

Cuisinart provided the Cuisinart Elite Collection 12 Cup food processor that was used for recipe testing in the book. This indispensable kitchen appliance came in handy for our entrées and desserts. *www.cuisinart.ca*

Eden Foods donated canned and dried beans, seaweed, soba noodles and other gourmet delights for recipe testing. We chose Eden canned beans because they have no salt added and have no BPA in the can linings. Thanks to Jonathan Wilson. *www.edenfoods.com*

Jensen Cheese and the **Wilton Cheese Factory** supplied us with outstanding quality colby and cheddar cheeses that are rennet-free with no added preservatives. Thank you to Eric and Scott Jensen, third-generation cheesemakers. *www.jensencheese.ca*

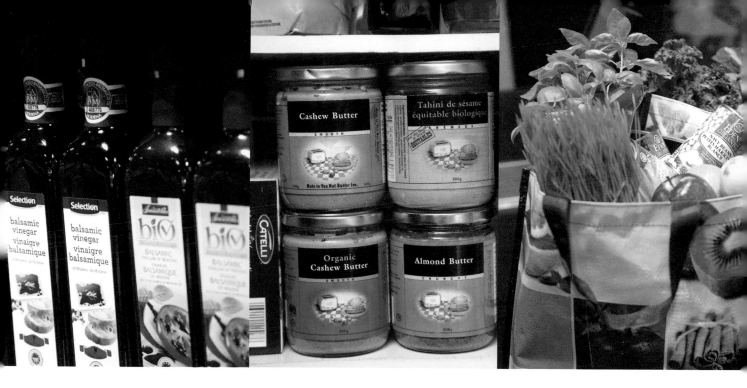

MacKellar Farms provided us with organic, non-GMO edamame, which grows locally in Ontario. They donated both in-shell and shelled edamame for recipe testing. Thanks to Jacob MacKellar for the fresh edamame too! *www.mackellarfarms.ca*

Maison Orphée supplied us with the best quality olive, canola and coconut oils, plus vinegar, sea salt and mustards. Thanks to Nathalie Plamondon and Sophie Larin. *www.maisonorphee.com*

Manitoba Harvest Hemp Foods supplied us with the best quality hemp seeds. *www.manitobaharvest.com*

Metro grocery stores donated their private label LifeSmart products for recipe testing and allowed us access to a Metro grocery store to capture beautiful photographs. Thanks to Jocelyne Martineau and Nancy Modrcin. *www.metro.ca*

Nuts to You donated products from their line of almond, cashew, peanut and tahini butters. Thanks to Sam Abrams, Kathleen Corrigan and Anne Lawrence. *www.nutstoyounutbutter.com*

Oldways, a US-based non-profit nutrition organization, gave us permission to use the Mediterranean Diet Pyramid that they created. Thanks to Rachel Greenstein. *www.oldwayspt.org*

Peanut Bureau of Canada helped feed our need for peanut butter, shell peanuts and roasted peanuts. Thanks to Kyla Best. *www.peanutbureau.ca*

Peter Piper Pepper supplied us with organic, fair trade tamari. Thanks to Gary Fenske and Christopher Jared. *www.jaredpacific.com*

Stonemill Bakehouse donated loaves of whole grain bread for recipe testing. Thanks to Gottfried Boehringer and Sloane Levitt. *www.stonemillbakehouse.com*

USA Rice Federation provided us with the highest quality short- and long-grain brown rice grown in the United States. Thanks to Pereina Choudhury. *www.riceinfo.com*

Zwilling J.A. Henckels provided our knives and other kitchen tools. Plus, their bamboo cutting boards, stainless steel whisks, pots and pans were useful for properly testing recipes. *www.zwilling.ca*

Thank You

From Cara

Thank you to my supportive, creative and wonderful friends: Daniella, Anthony, Erynn, Sari, James, Kim, Louise and Robin, who didn't mind asking the same question all year long: "How's the book going?"

Thanks to Kyle and Adi for farm-fresh maple syrup and perfect wooden serving boards.

Lots of gratitude goes to my fellow dietitians (too many to list!). Your words of wisdom, enticing recipes and passion for food keep me educated, inspired and well-nourished.

I could not have written this book without the help of my taste-testers, better known as my family: the ever-supportive Scott, Kasey, Aubrey and my dad, Jerry.

Thanks to my in-laws, Maxine and Harvey, who let us make a huge mess in their amazing kitchen, which was the perfect spot for recipe testing.

A special thanks to my niece Jess, whose inspiring courage always pushes me to do my very best.

From Nettie

Thank you to my ever-present, supportive friends: Barbara Barron, David Bird, Jocie Bussin, Marilyn Crowley, Alison Fryer, Naji Harb, Judi Schwartz and Mary Sharpe.

And thank you to my family: Helen Cronish, Sari Cronish, Suzie Siegal and my children, Cameron, Mackenzie and Emery Urquhart. And last, but never least, my wonderful husband, Jim.

Together, Cara and Nettie would like to thank:

- The team at Metro: Nancy Mordcin, Anna Pizyo-Way, Kayla Martins, Jocelyne Martineau, Kathleen O'Hara and Michelle Rowlands.

- The team at Whitecap: Nick Rundall, Jesse Marchand, Michelle Furbacher, Jordie Yow, Steph Hill, Patrick Geraghty, Maxine Matishak and Jacqueline Gubiani.

- Heather Howe, PHEc, recipe tester. Thanks for your ideas and expertise, which helped make our recipes perfect. But even more, thanks for being so easy to work with and such a pleasure to talk to and spend time with. *www.livintocook.ca*

- Amy Whitson, PHEc, nutrient analysis. Thank you for agreeing to do the nutrient analysis for 100 recipes with a newborn in tow! Your helpful notes, excellent feedback and keen eye helped us create something we are proud of. *www.thetk.ca*

- Jesse Blinick, lawyer at Blinick Law. Thanks for your patience and attention to detail. *www.blinicklaw.com*

- Gina St. Germain, Food and Prop Stylist. With your amazing sense of style, you created landscapes so our recipes could tell a story. And you do have the perfect dish for every picture! Thanks for your creative spirit and positive energy.

- Mike McColl, photographer. Wow. You took our recipes and turned them into works of art. Your creativity and vision were so appreciated. Thank you also Mia Bachmaier and Lee Waddington for your assistance.

Index